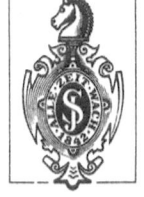

D. A. Buxton Hopkin

# Hazards and Errors in Anaesthesia

Springer-Verlag
Berlin Heidelberg New York 1980

D. A. Buxton Hopkin, MD, FFARCS

Honorary Consultant Anaesthetist
Charing Cross and St. Thomas' Hospitals and Medical
Schools
University of London

11 Chelsea Embankment
London SW3 4LE England

ISBN-13:978-3-540-10158-1     e-ISBN-13:978-1-4471-1298-3
DOI:10.1007/978-1-4471-1298-3

Library of Congress Cataloging in Publication Data. Hopkin, Denis Arthur
Buxton. Hazards and errors in anaesthesia. Bibliography: p. Includes index.
1. Anesthesia—Complications and sequelae. I. Title. II. Title: Errors in
anaesthesia. [DNLM: 1. Accident prevention. 2. Anesthesia—Adverse effects.
WO245 H793h] RD82.5.H66 617'.96 80-18942

2128/3916-543210

*To my wife*

# Contents

**Part IV   Individual Types of Procedure**

# Preface

This book has a twofold purpose, first to provide information for beginners about the pitalls and hazards of anaesthesia and second to help the occasional anaesthetist in remote areas when confronted with requests to anaesthetise for unfamiliar surgical operations.

The book is not intended to replace any standard text for anaesthetic examinations, and indeed, its lack of information about basic sciences makes it unsuitable for such a purpose.

The contents can be regarded as a distillate of 45 years of practical anaesthesia, in both primitive and sophisticated conditions, from the ether and chloroform rag and bottle days onwards through cyclopropane, trichloroethylene, relaxants and lytic cocktails to halothane. The only operation mentioned of which I have no practical experience is thymectomy and removal of an argentaffinoma. I have never knowingly encountered malignant hyperpyrexia, but had one experience of what we called ether convulsions with hyperpyrexia, which could have been, and probably was, the same thing.

An attempt has been made to arrange the book in four logical sections. It begins with the hazards of preparation—assessment of risks to patients particularly, but Part I also includes chapters on medicolegal and occupational hazards to anaesthetists.

Part II deals with the performance of anaesthesia and related matters that are relevant to all surgical procedures. As many anaesthetic accidents arise from faulty connections or from disconnections, a chapter is devoted to the care and preparation of anaesthetic apparatus and the need for systematic checking before use. Intensive care receives attention only insofar as concerns treatment of the respiratory distress syndrome and the ethics of organ transplantation, with which beginners and anaesthetists in isolated areas may find themselves involved.

Part III deals with anaesthesia for emergency surgery. This short section includes a chapter on shock states which is an attempt to simplify a subject which has become unnecessarily complicated over the years. Application of the views put forward could be very rewarding.

Part IV contains thumbnail sketches of operations by specialities and the anaesthetic problems to which they give rise and how they can be dealt with. It is by no means comprehensive and only intends to cover the conditions commonly encountered in everyday hospital practice. It does, however, include chapters on anaesthesia for day surgery and in radiological and cardiological departments.

Detailed references have been intentionally left out of the text, but at the end of the book a certain number of bibliographical references on selected subjects are listed, for those seeking further details. I hope they will be useful.

The suggestion that there was a need for a book such as this came from the late Paul B. Mayer, the London representative of Springer-Verlag, who himself experienced anaesthesia on more than one occasion during his last illness. Although seldom free from pain and progressively disabled he took an active interest in the project and his enthusiasm was a great stimulus. During his last days he continued to carry out his normal daily routine. His courage and fortitude evoked the admiration of everyone and I much regret he was unable to see the completed manuscript.

The onerous task of typing and retyping the manuscript was undertaken by Miss Elizabeth Mitchell, Secretary of the Anaesthetic Department at Charing Cross Hospital; by Miss Mary McRedmond, Miss Vanessa Rose and Miss Jane Fraser, members of Mrs Van Aernsbergen's Department of Secretarial Services, also at Charing Cross Hospital; and by Mrs Hettie Jones and Miss Clover Bygraves of West London Hospital. Each devoted many hours of spare time to typing and I thank them all.

The Department of Medical Illustration at Charing Cross Hospital Medical School undertook the redrawing and preparation for reproduction of Figs. 1, 2 and 5, and Mrs S. Godbolt and her staff at the Medical School Library checked the details of the bibliography. I am much indebted to all concerned.

Finally, it is a pleasure to acknowledge the help received from Mr Michael Jackson, Medical Editor of Springer-Verlag, and Mr Bruce Cameron, Copy Editor, whose advice and expertise have proved invaluable in deciding the final arrangement of the material, which Mr Roger Dobbing, Production Editor, and The Lavenham Press have produced so elegantly.

London, July 1980                                        D. A. Buxton Hopkin

# Part I

*Pre-operative Assessment,*
*Medicolegal and*
*Occupational Hazards*

# 1 General Considerations

Pre-operative assessment of patients for elective surgery, although acknowledged to be essential for planning safe anaesthesia and successful surgery, is too often perfunctory and carried out too late to be of any practical value. There are many reasons for this, including an excessively rapid turnover of patients in the interest of high bed occupancy, combined with a shortage of trained anaesthetists. Surgeons also carry some responsibility as improved safety of anaesthesia has encouraged concentration on the technical aspects of surgery without equal concern for the physical state of patients. Anaesthetists should never be hurried into anaesthetising badly prepared or unassessed patients in response to a request by surgical colleagues for a short anaesthetic. Too often the operation develops into a major procedure accompanied by complications due to lack of preparation and causes considerable anxiety to the anaesthetist.

It has often been said (referring to heavy smokers and drinkers) that the day before a major surgical operation is a poor time to change the habits of a lifetime. The same thought applies to pre-operative assessment: the night before a major operation is not the best time to carry it out. It is true that constant efforts are being made to ensure that anaesthetists have time to examine and assess their patients some days before the actual surgery, and the idea of anaesthetic assessment clinics where patients can be seen well in advance of their operation has much support. Although the proposal is excellent in theory, there are administrative problems and it is unlikely to be adopted widely until there are more anaesthetists available. Nevertheless, much can be achieved by close co-operation in hospitals between the surgical and anaesthetic residents. Surgical residents who know the schedules can often pass on advance information to their anaesthetic colleagues through the nursing staff. Whatever system is being followed, anaesthetists should have a planned procedure aimed at eliminating unforeseen complications, anticipating difficulties and allowing a reasonable assessment of risk, which may have to be set against the degree of seriousness or urgency of the proposed operation. Apart from their clinical value, recording these facts and findings is of increasing medicolegal importance and provides often the best protection against litigation to do with the anaesthetic which may arise after the operation. Many anaesthetists in the United States, where litigation has reached serious proportions, besides recording the pre-operative findings of all patients, include the technique they propose to use, with the reasons for their choice, as a protection against any subsequent medicolegal problems.

As in any other branch of medicine, the patient's history is of prime importance and a few moments spent on it can be rewarding. Apart from details of social habits, e.g. smoking and alcohol, and details of past and present operations, references to previous history of medical treatment, particularly of cardiovascular and respiratory ailments, and of any drug treatment prescribed either in the past or currently are very relevant. Increasing awareness of potential anaesthetic hazards of drug therapy has resulted in several hospitals issuing patients with a routine enquiry form about past and present drug therapy for their personal physician to complete and send to the hospital before their admission. All patients undergoing major surgery—or, in the opinion of many, any surgery—should have the following examination carried out in advance: (1) weight in kilograms, blood pressure, pulse and respiration rate; (2) chest X-ray; (3) if over 60, an ECG examination; (4) full blood count and, where appropriate, sickle test; (5) examination of urine for sugar, albumin and cellular deposits. Results of these investigations should be available at least 24 h before surgery. They should reveal any pathological conditions likely to constitute an added risk and allow time for their correction.

# 2 Cardiovascular Disease

Abnormalities of the cardiovascular system are encountered more frequently than any other defect. Long-standing cardiovascular disease is usually evident from the history or physical examination of the patient. Signs of untreated cardiac failure (orthopnoea, pulmonary congestion, enlarged heart, tender liver, rapid and irregular pulse) are absolute contra-indications for elective or emergency surgery. The assistance of a cardiologist should be sought and surgery postponed until the cardiac failure is under control. Statistics have shown that in these circumstances delay does not increase the overall mortality and, if anything, will decrease it.

## 2.1 Valvular Disease

Treated valvular disease where there is no failure is not a great added risk. Patients who have had repeated attacks of congestive failure, suggesting progressive reduction of cardiac reserve, are poor risks and unsuitable for major radical surgery. Patients with mitral valve disease, even if auricular fibrillation is present, tolerate major surgery very well. On the other hand, those with aortic valve disease, whether stenosis or regurgitation, stand anaesthesia very badly. In aortic valve disease the coronary arteries are always affected and there is a reduction in the amount of blood which the heart muscle can receive. Therefore, any additional strain on the heart muscle is likely to result in failure, since output is limited and a small fall of blood pressure, which often accompanies induction with barbiturates, can reduce coronary perfusion and oxygen supply to the already hypertrophied heart muscle. On the other hand, stimulation under light anaesthesia can lead to a rise in systolic blood pressure, increasing the work of the heart, for which adequate oxygen supplies are not available. Therefore, prognosis of aortic disease is poor at the best of times. The presence of cardiac asthma (nocturnal dyspnoea) implies a survival of less than 6 months and is always a contra-indication for anaesthesia, except for life-saving emergency operations.

## 2.2  Hypertension and Cardiac Ischaemia

Advances in treatment of hypertension and associated cardiac ischaemia have greatly improved expectation of life and patients under treatment present for assessment of anaesthetic risk in ever increasing numbers.

Often routine blood pressure measurements before operation reveal unexpectedly high figures in newly admitted patients, in spite of there being no previous history. High readings can arise from apprehension, and measurements made a few hours later will usually be within normal limits.

### 2.2.1  Management of Patients Receiving Antihypertensive Drugs

Patients with established hypertensive disease are usually under treatment with a beta-adrenergic receptor blocker (propranolol); a blocker of adrenergic neuronal transmission (guanethidine); or agents which interfere with synthesis of noradrenaline, such as methyldopa (Aldomet), whose inhibition of decarboxylase prevents conversion of naturally occurring L-dopa to dopamine, itself a precursor of nor-adrenaline.

When these drugs were first introduced for treatment of hypertension, many anaesthetists felt that the administration of anaesthetics (all of which lower blood pressure) to patients receiving them was unjustifiable, owing to the risk of inducing catastrophic falls in systolic blood pressure, which would endanger cerebral and coronary circulation. Many anaesthetists insisted on discontinuation of therapy for 14 days before elective surgery, during which the cardiac and cerebral symptoms which had led the patient to seek medical advice often returned.

This practice was unpopular with patients and their practitioners and it is now agreed there is no need to stop antihypertensive treatment before anaesthesia. Clinical observations have established that untreated patients and those whose therapy has been discontinued tolerate anaesthesia and surgery less well than those who are under treatment with antihypertensive agents.

### 2.2.2  Factors Increasing Myocardial Ischaemia

Electrocardiographic signs of myocardial ischaemia (flattened S-T segment), often accompanied by marked increase in blood pressure brought about by an increase of adrenergic activity, have been observed in the course of:

1) Laryngoscopy and endotracheal intubation

2) Bronchoscopy or tracheal suction

3) Surgical incision

4) Traction on mesentery during routine laparotomy

5) Clamping of aorta during arterial surgery

6) Recovery, when pain sensation and central autonomic reflexes return and induce increase of adrenergic activity

In patients who are not receiving treatment these episodes of high blood pressure place an added burden on heart muscle. The greater tension of cardiac muscle required to overcome the enhanced peripheral resistance increases the demand for oxygen, which the impaired coronary circulation finds difficulty in meeting. On the other hand, patients whose antihypertensive therapy has not been interrupted show fewer signs of physiological disturbance during anaesthesia and surgery.

Practical experience confirms these findings. Patients with renal disease, although always receiving high dosage of beta blocking agents, tolerate general anaesthesia very well and no reports have appeared of severe reduction of blood pressure.

Cautious anaesthetists are warned against arriving at a compromise by reducing the dose of antihypertensive medication before anaesthesia. This will only create an unstable condition, and hypertensive episodes during surgery will increase in number and be comparable in severity to those encountered in untreated patients.

## 2.3  Coronary Artery Disease, Angina and Myocardial Infarction

The presence of evidence of coronary artery disease increases the overall mortality during or following surgical procedures, but the time interval between infarction and surgery and the type of infarct, whether transmural or subendocardial, also have considerable influence on the prognosis.

### 2.3.1  Operative Mortality

When 4 months has passed since the infarction, the postoperative mortality is half that of patients who have suffered infarct recently (i.e. less than 3 months before operation), but it is about twice that of patients with no evidence of coronary artery disease. After 6 months, operative mortality falls to 5%, which is a little higher than the overall average. However, there is a strongly held view in Great Britain that the mortality after 6 months does not differ significantly from that of patients who have not had infarct.

The outlook for patients who have had a transmural infarction is much poorer than for those with subendocardial lesions, the mortality for patients with transmural lesions being ten times greater. It has often been suggested that older patients (aged 70 or more) are less liable to postoperative infarction than younger ones since sufferers from serious coronary disease seldom survive beyond 65 years. Figures published in the United States do not support this idea and indicate that the risk is nearly doubled.

### 2.3.2  Myocardial Infarction During Anaesthesia

Infarction during anaesthesia must be extremely rare. It has occurred during procedures under local analgesia in an apprehensive and inadequately sedated patient and in a patient undergoing dental extraction under hypoxic nitrous oxide. Sedation for patients with a history of infarction who are to undergo procedures under local or regional anaesthesia should include strong tranquillising agents— droperidol, promazine or chlorpromazine—as well as opiates and beta-adrenergic blockers.

### 2.3.3  Anaesthetic Management

When general anaesthesia is to be employed attention should be directed to choice of techniques that allow liberal supplies of oxygen whilst allowing maintenance of a depth of anaesthesia sufficient to subdue adrenergic response to surgical stimulation and ensure a gradual return to consciousness. Rapid recovery and inadequate postoperative control of pain are not in the best interest of patients with a history of infarction. Some workers recommend a small intravenous injection of an opiate (e.g. 25 mg pethidine) as the procedure is ending to ensure freedom from pain during the early recovery phase. Although the incidence of post-operative infarction is not high (5%), the mortality when infarction does occur is very high, averaging 54%. These considerations underline the importance of a pre-operative ECG in all patients over 60, as well as a careful enquiry into the history behind any positive finding. Although the patient may be symptom-free at the time of examination, a pre-operative ECG, whether normal or abnormal, serves as a baseline for comparison with any postoperative ECG taken in connection with the diagnosis of postoperative complications.

### 2.3.4  Undiagnosed Myocardial Infarction

Although fatal infarction during anaesthesia is not widely reported, the author has on two occasions anaesthetised patients who suffered a fatal but silent infarction 24-48 h before anaesthesia and surgery. Absence of signs of cardiac failure or complaint of distress explains the failure to diagnose the condition. One patient died 12 h and the other 48 h after operation. At post-mortem in both cases necrosis of left ventricular muscle was present. One of the patients had myocardial disease of several years standing and complained of transient angina pain 36 h before surgery; the pain responded to rest and analgesics. The other suffered a hypotensive episode 36-48 h before operation. This was thought by the intern to be a small gastric haemorrhage and was one of the reasons for advancing the time of surgery and for the failure to take an ECG before anaesthesia.

# 3 Respiratory Disease

## 3.1  Common Cold

Complications of the common cold, particularly tracheitis, are indications for postponement of elective major surgery. Infection can easily spread from the upper respiratory tract into the lungs after autonomic disturbance during surgery. Animal experimentation undertaken some years ago showed that irritation of autonomic nerve endings in the pharynx can induce hyperaemia of the lungs; this in its turn attracted pathogenic organisms previously placed in mediastinal lymph nodes and which hitherto had remained inactive.

## 3.2  Chronic Respiratory Disease

When pre-operative clinical examination shows evidence of respiratory disease, elective operations should be delayed to allow assessment of lung function and institution of measures to improve it. Sophisticated equipment is not necessary and tests can be made at the bedside.

### 3.2.1  Vitalograph

Measurement of forced expiratory volume in 1 s ($FEV_1$) and forced vital capacity (FVC) can be made with the Vitalograph, which consists of a bag attached to a device into which patients make maximum expiration. The required data is presented in graphic form which patients can see. In normal subjects the ratio between $FEV_1$ and FVC should be around 80%. Figures of 60% or less indicate impaired function and treatment is needed. The Vitalograph has the advantage of allowing patients to see the results of their tests and of the improvement that breathing exercises and giving up smoking can bring about. In this way, patients are more co-operative and better results are obtained.

### 3.2.2  Peak Flow Meter
The Wright peak flow meter is another simple device to measure patients' expiratory gas flow rate. The lower limit of normal is 350 l/min; anything less indicates a need for pre-operative therapy.

### 3.2.3  Match and Breath-Holding Tests
If measuring equipment is unavailable, the match and breath-holding tests are two good ways of assessing respiratory function. The match test involves extinguishing in one breath a lighted match held 7-8 cm from the open mouth; failure indicates maximum breathing capacity is only 50% of normal. Alternatively, patients who cannot hold their breath for 25 s following full inspiration also have reduced breathing capacity of about 50%.

## 3.3  Methods of Improving Lung Function

Breathing exercises, giving up smoking and, if sputum is plentiful, postural drainage and bronchodilator drugs will help improve lung function. If sputum culture reveals pathogenic organisms, appropriate antibiotics should be started. Aminophylline and salbutamol help to lessen the tenacity of the sputum and any bronchospasm. Inhalation of aromatic agents, e.g. friar's balsam in boiling water, is an excellent alternative.

## 3.4  Anaesthetic Management

Patients with diseased lungs can be classified roughly into three categories:

1) Persistent cough and sputum, respiratory function tests within normal limits and normal chest X-ray. Anaesthetic hazards are minimal and no reason exists for delay of operation. Postoperative chest physiotherapy is advisable after upper abdominal surgery.

2) Persistent cough and sputum, reduced lung function ($FEV_1$:FVC below 60%), breathlessness on exertion, but normal blood gases. Patients should have pre-operative chest physiotherapy and antibiotics 24 h before operation and continued afterwards.

3) Patients are breathless at rest, unable to lie flat and sleep in the sitting position. Blood gases abnormal ($PaO_2$ below 9.3 kPa). Careful

pre-operative preparation is called for as in category 2, and after upper abdominal or thoracic surgery mechanical ventilation will probably be required for 24-48 h. Patients with extensive respiratory disease tolerate major surgery surprisingly well. Recent advances in intensive care and mechanical support by ventilators, facilities for estimation of blood gases and improvements in nursing care and physiotherapy have all made significant contributions.

### 3.4.1 Premedication
Respiratory depressants should be avoided in favour of drugs which reduce secretions and spasm. Atropine or any of the phenothiazine derivatives is useful.

### 3.4.2 Anaesthetic Techniques
Extensive pulmonary disease is an indication for regional, subdural or epidural methods (see Chap. 17).

General anaesthetic techniques vary with the operation. Many anaesthetistis include 40-60 mg gallamine (Flaxedil) in 0.5 g thiopentone to avoid the coughing which often accompanies induction of anaesthesia in chronic bronchitic patients. If intubation is necessary, thiopentone induction followed by spraying of the cords and trachea with 4% lignocaine together with a rapid-acting relaxant provides an opportunity to introduce a sufficient concentration of non-irritant inhalational agents to suppress respiratory irritability before spontaneous breathing returns. Trichloroethylene does not reduce bronchial irritability and should be avoided in bronchitic patients.

Large doses of relaxants are not necessary for upper abdominal surgery in chronic bronchitics. Abdominal muscle tone is usually poor in such patients and if large doses of relaxants are given, problems may arise in their reversal (see Sect. 13.1.6).

## 3.5 Asthma

Asthmatic patients are usually in category 2. The principles for treatment mentioned above apply, but careful attention should be given to choice of a suitable time for operation when climatic and physical conditions are favourable. The anaesthetic techniques do not differ from those outlined. It should be remembered that asthmatic patients often receive steroid treatment (see Sect. 7.1) and enquiries should always precede any anaesthetic or operation.

# 4 Haematological Disorders

## 4.1  Anaemia

Asymptomatic anaemia is not rare, but it is often only revealed after routine pre-anaesthetic examination. Continued intermittent bleeding from chronic menorrhagia in women, or from haemorrhoids in either sex, is a common cause. Malnutrition is also a factor in elderly people who live alone.

Haemoglobin values below 10 g/100 ml are usually regarded as a contra-indication to elective major surgery, since a low level of haemoglobin is associated with a higher incidence of postoperative complications than is observed in subjects with normal values.

Corrective measures for anaemia depend upon the cause, the severity and the extent of the proposed surgical procedure.

### 4.1.1  Iron Deficiency Anaemia

When surgery is not urgent, iron deficiency anaemia from chronic haemorrhage or dietary deficiency can be corrected with iron therapy and vitamin supplements over 2 weeks. If surgery cannot be delayed, pre-operative transfusion should be arranged, but since the anaemia is 'compensated' (i.e. the blood volume is normal) care should be taken to avoid overloading the circulation. Slow transfusion of packed cells on the day before operation avoids this hazard.

### 4.1.2  Anaemia Due to Chronic Renal Failure or Sickle-Cell Disease

Patients with chronic renal failure or sickle-cell disease have permanent anaemia, which is well compensated, and transfusion is not required for minor surgical procedures. The fact that cyanosis does not appear until the level of circulating haemoglobin in reduced form reaches 5 g/100 ml is a major hazard of severe anaemia. Cyanosis in a patient with a haemoglobin level of 7 or 8 g/100 ml indicates a potentially fatal hypoxia. Cyanosis should never be allowed to occur in anaemic patients.

### 4.1.3  Megaloblastic Anaemias

Pernicious anaemia is typical megaloblastic anaemia and is controlled by liver and folic acid.

Megaloblastic anaemia also occurs in sufferers from myxoedema, in alcoholics with a dietary folic acid deficiency, following continued ingestion of contraceptive pills containing oestrogen, and after long-term treatment with psychotropic drugs such as phenytoin and phenobarbitone for treatment of epilepsy.

Megaloblastic anaemia also occurs in sufferers from liver disease.

Correction of anaemia with liver extracts and folic acid should be undertaken before elective surgery. When surgery is urgent, transfusion of packed cells should be arranged before operation.

Since megaloblastic anaemias are sometimes associated with a neurological disorder, epidural and subdural techniques are best avoided in those affected.

## 4.2  Polycythaemia Rubra Vera

Polycythaemia is a neoplastic condition of red and white blood cells. Patients appear in good health with a highly coloured complexion but feel unwell. The associated increase in the volume and viscosity of the blood places a severe strain on the cardiovascular system and increases the hazards of major surgery.

Haemoconcentration must be avoided at all costs during surgery. Blood loss should be accurately replaced by electrolyte solutions to reduce viscosity. In polycythaemia patients the reduced perfusion accompanying vasoconstriction due to shock carries a real danger of infarction and thrombosis.

Vasodilator inhalational anaesthetics such as halothane help to dilate small vessels and improve perfusion. If blood viscosity produces signs of left ventricular failure, venesection of 500 ml blood and replacement by isotonic electrolyte solutions will improve cardiac function.

## 4.3 Leukaemia

Acute leukaemia is often rapidly fatal and patients seldom present for anaesthesia and surgery. The associated thrombocytopenia increases liability to haemorrhage after trauma and should need arise for anaesthesia, care and gentleness during endotracheal intubation are essential and it should be avoided if possible.

Chronic leukaemia patients are usually receiving steroids and cytotoxic drugs. Before anaesthesia, steroid replacement therapy with hydrocortisone is essential (see Sect. 7.1). Patients receiving cytotoxic drugs will have low white cell counts and prophylactic broad spectrum antibiotics are required before surgery, in view of such patients' lowered resistance to infection. Anaemia may need correction, and thrombocytopenia is an indication for infusion of fresh blood or platelets before any operation.

## 4.4 Multiple Myeloma

Myeloma is a malignant proliferation of plasma cells in the form of small tumours in bone marrow. Symptoms arise from pathological fractures, from pressure on nerves and nerve roots, and depression of blood formation. Handling of such patients presents a very real hazard on the operating table and gentleness is essential to avoid pathological fractures. Compression fractures of vertebral bodies may result in paraplegia. Fracture of the ribs will restrict breathing and cause postoperative pulmonary complications.

## 4.5 Haemorrhagic Disorders

Unexpected haemorrhage during and immediately after surgical operations, not arising directly from the procedure itself, occurs from deficiency in platelets (thrombocytopenia) and of substances necessary for coagulation, such as fibrinogen, prothrombin and factor VIII (haemophilia and Christmas disease).

The conditions can often be anticipated and corrected before anaesthesia and surgery. They can also occur spontaneously during major surgical procedures associated with severe haemorrhage of following cardiopulmonary by-pass.

### 4.5.1 Thrombocytopenia

Thrombocytopenia, or platelet deficiency, can occur idiopathically. It is also associated with other conditions: leukaemia, aplastic anaemia, advanced liver disease, scurvy and severe virus disease or bacterial infections.

Excessive bleeding during operation can be expected when platelet counts fall below $50\,000/mm^3$. Pre-operative infusion of a platelet concentrate is essential. If unavailable, whole blood transfusion is an acceptable substitute.

### 4.5.2 Haemophilia and Christmas Disease

Haemophilia and the closely related Christmas disease are male sex-linked hereditary diseases transmitted by females. Either factor VIII or factor IX or Christmas factor, which resembles factor VII, necessary for blood clotting, is absent. Diagnosis is often delayed until suggested by excessive bleeding or bruising following a minor surgical procedure such as dental extraction or after mild trauma. Once diagnosed, sufferers attend a haemophilia centre where the extent of the factor deficiency and the amount required before surgery is estimated. This information is entered on a 'haemophilia card' issued to patients which they should always carry. Before any anaesthetic or surgical procedure the patients must receive the quantity of factor VIII indicated on the card in the form of cryoprecipitate concentrate. If that is not available, an acceptable alternative is fresh whole blood or fresh frozen plasma concentrate together with aminocaproic acid, which hinders lysis of blood clots.

Cryoprecipitate is stored frozen in plastic bags containing 20-30 ml plasma. After thawing in a water bath at 37°C and squeezing several times to dissolve the precipitate, the contents of the bag can be introduced through an intravenous drip or injected directly from a syringe. The recommended dose is 2 units/12 kg body weight, 1 h before operation, followed by half this amount every 12 h for 2 or 3 days after operation, since the half-life of factor VIII does not exceed 12 h.

### 4.5.3 Anaesthetic Management

Special precautions are recommended to prevent haemorrhagic complications when it is known in advance that a patient suffers from haemophilia or purpura:

1) Intramuscular injections should be avoided completely because they may induce the formation of a haematoma. Premedication should be given by mouth or by the intravenous route.

2) Endotracheal intubation should only be undertaken when really necessary and then only after full muscle relaxation. During exposure of the larynx minimal pressure on the tongue and fauces is necessary to avoid haemorrhage or haematoma formation. Nasal intubation should never be attempted because it could lead to copious haemorrhage.

3) Intravenous induction is safe if a very small gauge needle is used, but many anaesthetists prefer to rely on inhalational anaesthetic techniques.

4) Regional methods are of course contra-indicated.

### 4.5.4  Dental Extraction on Haemophilic Patients

To avoid troublesome haemorrhage after dental extractions, the patient should receive a transfusion of cryoprecipitate on the morning of operation sufficient to bring factor VIII concentration up to 50% of normal, followed by epsilon-aminocaproic acid 0.1 g/kg i.v. to stabilise clot formation and delay its destruction.

Administration of epsilon-aminocaproic acid can be continued afterwards by mouth four times a day for a week. Postoperative aspirin to control pain is contra-indicated because it can cause gastro-intestinal haemorrhage.

### 4.5.5  Anticoagulant Therapy

Patients often receive small doses of heparin with the object of reducing deep vein thrombosis after operation. Small doses are said not to increase operative bleeding, but blood loss from postoperative oozing is often greater than normal. A wise precaution is to estimate the pro-thrombin level before major procedures. If this is not below 20% of normal it is safe to proceed with surgery.

During major arterial and open-heart surgery, patients receive large doses of heparin; these should be neutralised at the end of the operation by administration of protamine sulphate.

### 4.5.6  Fibrinolysis

Abnormal bleeding during major procedures from deficient blood clotting sometimes occurs in patients who have had multiple blood transfusions or who have undergone more than one operation within a short time. Precise definition of the clotting defect requires full haemato-logical examination, for which there is no time, as immediate action is required. The condition arises from deficiency in fibrin or lack of platelets. The best treatment is infusion of fresh frozen plasma, which is twice as effective as whole blood for replacement of clotting factors. Initially an infusion of 1 litre over 1 h is recommended to replace the lost factors, and 1 litre every 12 h thereafter until bleeding is controlled.

## 4.6  Sickle-Cell Disease

Sickle-cell anaemia or haemoglobin S disease is mainly confined to negro races, but it is also found amongst the indigenous inhabitants of parts of Greece, Asia Minor and northern India.

Red blood cells of such persons contain an abnormal haemoglobin, haemoglobin S, which, when deprived of oxygen, crystallises inside the red cell producing the deformity known as sickling. This in turn causes rupture, blocking and damage to capillaries.

A positive sickle-cell test indicates the presence of the trait and the need for further investigation by electrophoresis to determine whether it is homozygous or heterozygous.

The *homozygous* trait is the more dangerous. The blood of such patients may contain as much as 90% abnormal haemoglobin. Sickling occurs at an oxygen tension as high as 5.3 kPa, equivalent to that of mixed venous blood, so that destruction of red cells is constantly occurring and the patients are always anaemic.

The blood of *heterozygous* patients, on the other hand, does not carry more than 40% of abnormal haemoglobin. Sickling does not take place until oxygen tension in the blood falls to 2.7 kPa, a figure well below that of mixed venous blood. The main hazard in such patients is lack of oxygen during or after anaesthesia and surgery, which will precipitate sickling and subsequent complications.

### 4.6.1  Pre-anaesthetic Management

Patients who ethnologically are potential sickle trait carriers should be screened before anaesthesia as part of the routine haemoglobin and blood estimation. For emergencies, a 'do-it-yourself' kit, known as Sickledex, is available and should be standard equipment in anaesthetic rooms. When the test is positive, electrophoresis is really necessary to determine the nature of the trait, but in emergency, microscopic examination of a blood film will show the presence or absence of red cell abnormalities. When the red cells are not abnormal it is reasonable to assume a heterozygous condition and proceed with anaesthesia and surgery with certain precautions. If there are abnormalities, and the patient is anaemic, the presence of the high-risk homozygous trait should be assumed and anaesthesia planned accordingly.

The use of a tourniquet is contra-indicated in all patients who suffer from sickle disease, for the obvious reason that the deprivation of oxygen which its application entails could easily start a sickling crisis.

*Heterozygous (Low-Risk) Trait.* Anaesthesia and surgery in the presence of heterozygous sickle trait are less hazardous than was at first thought. In Ghana, where the trait is common, patients tolerate anaesthesia and surgery well and complications are rare. However, any infections should be treated with antibiotics, and anaemia with iron or transfusion.

Anaesthetic techniques and premedication should avoid oxygen lack from respiratory depression and the use of opiates before or during operation is best avoided. Techniques should be simple but to ensure absolute freedom from respiratory obstruction, endotracheal intubation under full relaxation with suxamethonium is advised. At the end of operation anaesthesia should not be too light, so as to avoid a spasmodic episode and temporary hypoxia on extubation.

*Homozygous (High-Risk) Trait.* Anaesthesia and surgery should only be undertaken in patients with the homozygous trait after careful preparation. Any pre-existing infection should be cleared up and the patient brought to as good a physical condition as possible by transfusion of packed blood cells until the level of haemoglobin reaches 12 or 13 g/100 ml.

## 4.6.2 Anaesthetic Technique

The anaesthetic technique is the same for the two traits, except that, of course, in homozygous patients inspired oxygen concentration should never fall below 30% and indeed there is much to be said for giving 100% with an inhalational agent such as halothane or cyclopropane.

During operation any blood loss must be accurately replaced, and since repeated transfusions (which these patients always need) depress bone marrow function, slow transfusion should continue after operation for 24 h.

## 4.6.3 Postoperative Management

During recovery the patient should be nursed in the lateral position to avoid respiratory obstruction.

Energetic postoperative chest physiotherapy and early ambulation are essential to prevent chest infections and associated hypoxia, which can trigger a sickling crisis.

*Bone Marrow Infarction.* If bone pains occur, one should suspect infarction of bone marrow, a condition associated with a sickling crisis. This complication is so serious that suspicion alone is a sign for active treatment by heparin and magnesium sulphate. Alkalinisation of blood with sodium bicarbonate has been recommended to reduce the incidence of sickling. However, in spite of several trials no benefit has been established.

*Shock.* The histotoxic or stagnant anoxia which occurs during haemorrhagic or endotoxin shock is quite capable of triggering a sickling crisis. During recovery, estimations of blood $Pa_{O_2}$ are a helpful guide to any degree of hypoxia. Vasoconstriction, with cyanosis of nail beds or lips is another indication of peripheral hypoxia. Energetic measures should be taken to restore perfusion by any of the methods mentioned in Chap. 26.

## 4.7  Thalassaemia

Thalassaemia is a variety of sickle-cell disease occurring in inhabitants of
the eastern Mediterranean region (*thalassa* being Greek for sea), but it
also occurs in the Middle East and northern India. Patients may have one
of three abnormal haemoglobins: haemoglobin C, which gives a mild
form of thalassaemia; haemoglobin S, when it will resemble sickle
disease; and haemoglobin E, responsible for a severe form, thalassaemia
major. Sufferers often have mongoloid facies, which may serve as a
reminder of the condition.

### 4.7.1  Thalassaemia Major

Patients with thalassaemia major (Cooley's disease, Mediterranean
anaemia or target cell anaemia) are always anaemic and dependent on
blood transfusions. Continuous haemolysis results in hyperplasia of the
bone marrow with rarefaction of the long bones. Before anaesthesia and
surgery, a transfusion of packed cells is always necessary to bring
haemoglobin to at least 10 g/100 ml. Patients are liable to liver, renal or
left ventricular failure due to haemosiderosis, which is not always as
severe as in other haemolytic disease, however. Infections are common in
the presence of neutropenia and a low platelet count may cause
prolonged operative bleeding.

### 4.7.2  Thalassaemia Minor

Apart from having mild anaemia, patients with thalassaemia minor are
quite well. Anaemia is intensified during pregnancy or infection and
transfusion of packed cells will be required, certainly before surgery.
Indeed, it is said that blood transfusion is the lifeline of sufferers from
both types of thalassaemia.

# 5 Muscular Disorders

## 5.1 Myasthenia Gravis

Myasthenia gravis is an auto-immune disease characterised by a pro-nounced muscular weakness arising from a defect in transmission of nerve impulses at myoneural junctions. It resembles the action of curare and similar drugs. The similarity extends to the action of anticholin-esterase drugs, such as neostigmine, which reverse the muscle weakness arising from either cause. Myasthenic patients should never receive curare or drugs with a similar action. Such an eventuality is unlikely since the muscle weakness accompanying the disease makes muscle relaxants unnecessary.

Some myasthenic patients have tumours of the thymus gland, whose removal often results in improvement of the condition (details of this formidable operation are given in Sect. 42.5).

### 5.1.1 Premedication and Anaesthesia

Apart from the sensitivity to curare of myasthenic patients, the main risk of anaesthesia in patients with muscular dystrophies is the severe limitation of respiratory function which muscle weakness imposes.

Pre-operative assessment should include blood gas analysis, lung function tests and X-ray of the chest. After any operation, respiratory support by ventilator must be available and patients should be supervised in an intensive care unit for at least 24 h.

Opiate premedication is contra-indicated because the accompanying respiratory depression can precipitate respiratory failure.

Inhalation or intravenous anaesthetics are not contra-indicated, but only about half the quantity a normal patient would require is needed.

Postoperatively muscle weakness reduces ability to bring up secretions, and pulmonary complications after upper abdominal surgery are almost inevitable, often precipitating respiratory failure.

## 5.2  Myasthenic Syndrome

Some other diseases associated with muscle weakness resemble myasthenia gravis. They are difficult to recognise because they display the same response to curare. This occurs in patients with secondary deposits from carcinoma of the lung, in those receiving large doses of steroids and also in some dermatomyositis states.

It is possible to distinguish the two groups because true myasthenic patients, although sensitive to the action of curare and similar drugs, respond normally to depolarising agents such as suxamethonium. Those with a myasthenic syndrome, on the other hand, exhibit sensitivity to both types of relaxant.

## 5.3  Muscular Dystrophies

Anaesthesia is sometimes requested for patients suffering from a variety of rare and obscure muscular disorders, some of neurological origin, some of congenital origin, and others arising from old poliomyelitis. Nearly all have atrophy or weakness of the muscles or respiration and live on the brink of respiratory failure, which can be precipitated by a mild upper respiratory infection, by drugs which depress respiration or by an upper abdominal incision. The anaesthetic management of these patients differs in no way from that already described for myasthenia gravis patients.

## 5.4  Myotonia Congenita

Unlike the muscular dystrophies, which cause weakness, myotonia congenita is characterised by stiffness of muscles, which is accentuated by inactivity and cold.

Premedication and anaesthesia must be designed to avoid intensification of muscle stiffness, either with drugs, emotion or cold. Patients should be kept fairly warm and receive as premedication drugs that depress emotion and reduce muscle tone. Chlorpromazine possesses both these qualities and would be suitable. Since depolarising muscle relaxants cause muscle fasciculation and anticholinesterase intensifies stiffness, both should not be used.

Postoperative shivering can result in retraction of the chest and depression of respiration, as well as predisposing to hyperkalaemia. Again chlorpromazine would seem to have ideal properties for preventing these complications and its use, either as premedication or as part of the anaesthetic technique, appears logical.

# 6 Other Intercurrent Diseases

6.1 Diabetes
6.2 Obesity
6.3 Liver Disease
6.4 Kidney Disease

## 6.1 Diabetes

Sufferers from diabetes can be classified in three groups:

1) *Mild* diabetes can be controlled with diet and oral hypoglycaemic drugs. Anaesthesia and surgery carry little added risk. Oral hypoglycaemic therapy is omitted on the day of operation and resumed when the patient is able to take food again.

2) *More severe* diabetes requires insulin and diet for control. Anaesthesia and surgery carry little risk, but it is advisable for the anaesthetist and physician in charge of the patient to draw up an agreed plan of action based on the following principles: Ordinary insulin should be substituted for lente insulin on the day of operation in half the usual lente dose, together with 50 g glucose in the form of an intravenous 5% glucose infusion. Blood sugar estimations made before and after operation determine future requirements of insulin and glucose. Blood sugar estimation and urine testing for ketones should continue twice daily until patients are able to take a normal diet.

3) Patients with *uncontrolled* diabetes whose urine is loaded with sugar and contains acetone, who are receiving no treatment or in whom treatment has failed to control the illness, are in danger. The stress of surgery and anaesthesia can provoke a rise in blood sugar and precipitate diabetic coma. Anaesthesia is contra-indicated until administration of insulin and intravenous glucose and alkaline infusions have overcome acidosis and reduced blood sugar to a manageable level.

Degenerative arterial disease commonly accompanies diabetes. Before anaesthesia, careful assessment should be made of the cardiovascular system for signs of cardiac ischaemic disease.

Diabetic patients also suffer from neurological degenerative conditions affecting the autonomic as well as the peripheral nervous systems. In addition to foot-drop from peripheral neuritis, autonomic neuropathy can cause delayed emptying of the stomach and impaired vascular reflexes.

## 6.2  Obesity

Gross obesity has a reduced life expectancy in the view of most insurance companies. Obesity also presents special hazards in anaesthesia, those of a physical nature being almost as serious as those of a physiopathological nature.

In the course of pre-operative assessment, obese patients will be found to have a reduced vital capacity, often breathing only with the diaphragm ('belly breathing'). This results in under-ventilation of the lungs during anaesthesia and during recovery.

Ischaemic heart disease is not uncommon and blood volume may also be increased. Postoperative pulmonary complications and deep vein thrombosis are more frequent than in normal patients. Immobility after operation is a possible explanation.

The physical hazards associated with the bulk of obese patients and difficulties in airway maintenance also merit attention. Airway maintenance is complicated by the excess fat around and under the jaw presenting practical difficulties in locating the horizontal and vertical rami of the jaw and bringing it forwards to clear the airway. For this reason, for any but the shortest procedure, endotracheal intubation is desirable, and mechanical ventilation should continue for some hours after upper abdominal or thoracotomy operations.

Lifting very fat patients and settling them on the operating table also presents unusual problems. For instance for those weighing over 125 kg it is helpful to put two operating tables side by side. For lifting, four strong people should share the burden. Should it be necessary to turn patients into the lateral position, great care must be taken to prevent the patient falling off the table and again, at least two assistants in addition to the anaesthetist and a nurse should be available.

## 6.3  Liver Disease

Sufferers from liver disease present a wide range of hazards. Nutritional and drug metabolism is depressed, prolonging the action of barbiturates and potentiating the action of opiates to such a degree that a small dose of pethidine given to a patient on the brink of liver failure can induce a state of coma.

The depression of liver function also affects the power of the blood to form clots. The synthesis of prothrombin is depressed through delayed absorption of vitamin K (this is common even in obstructive jaundice) and even when vitamin K is available, damage to liver cells interferes with prothrombin formation. Hence, haemorrhage during operation and oozing after it can be expected.

Another liver function of considerable importance but often forgotten is the power to neutralise endotoxin. When liver function is depressed endotoxin neutralisation is reduced and the endotoxin titre in the blood rises. This has an adverse affect on kidney function and can often lead to renal failure. This is known as the hepatorenal syndrome.

Advanced cirrhotic disease presents hazards of haemorrhage from oesophageal varices, and operations to relieve congestion of the portal system are often required (see Chap. 29).

Patients with liver disease or jaundice should always receive vitamin K pre-operatively to ensure thrombin formation, and fresh frozen plasma should be available for treatment of coagulation deficiencies (see Sect. 4.5). Some units prescribe 20% mannitol in quantities of 200 ml and 50 ml during operation to improve urine output. Chlorpromazine antagonises endotoxin and reduces antidiuretic hormone secretion. Used with caution, it can be of value in these conditions.

## 6.4  Kidney Disease

Patients may present for anaesthesia with acute or chronic renal failure. Those with acute renal failure, whether it has arisen from 'shock' states or disease of the urinary tract, are usually in a state of metabolic acidosis requiring corrective treatment before induction of anaesthesia (see Sect. 27.3.3). Those in chronic renal failure are usually on dialysis, but may require anaesthesia for nephrectomy, insertion of shunts or renal transplantation. All are hypertensive and anaemic. Hypertension is controlled with antihypertensive drugs, whose administration should not be discontinued before anaesthesia.

Although anaemia is severe, compensatory increase in blood volume has taken place and transfusion is not necessary for short procedures. Conventional anaesthetic techniques using thiopentone, halothane, nitrous oxide and oxygen give good operating conditions, provided that the presence of anaemia is remembered and liberal supplies of oxygen made available. Hazards of anaesthesia for renal transplantation are considered in Sect. 32.2.

When anaesthesia is induced by intravenous injection in patients with chronic renal failure, the use of veins of the forearm, especially on the radial side, is forbidden. These veins in the proximity of the radial artery are reserved for the creation of shunts, without which satisfactory dialysis cannot be performed.

# 7 Adverse Reactions Due to Drug Therapy

7.1 **Steroids**
7.2 **Psychotropic Agents**
7.3 **Allergy**

Many therapeutic agents intensify the effects of anaesthetics or interfere with the response to surgery.

The same chemical compound assumes so many trade names that problems arise deciding to which class of compound it belongs. Hence before admission to hospital the patient receives a form for his or her personal physician to give details of any drugs which the patient has recently received, for inclusion in the hospital medical record.

Drugs with possible adverse affects during anaesthesia or surgery comprise: steroids and related compounds; psychotropic agents; and antihypertensive compounds (already discussed in Sect. 2.2.1).

## 7.1 Steroids

Steroid therapy is prescribed for arthritis, asthma, ulcerative colitis, Crohn's disease and chronic inflammatory conditions of the skin.

Prolonged treatment results in atrophy of the adrenal cortex, so that it becomes unable to produce glucocorticoids in response to infection, injury, haemorrhage or surgical trauma. After operation, such patients are liable to go into adrenal failure. The symptoms—asthenia, severe hypotension and reduction of blood sodium—can be confused with postoperative shock, with fatal results if corticoid therapy is not instituted.

Adrenal failure can be prevented by administering supplementary hydrocortisone pre-operatively to any patient who has received steroid therapy within the past 3 months.

Formerly it was taught that patients who at any time had been treated with steroids should always receive cover before operation. It is now known that if steroid therapy has been discontinued for more than 3 months, pre-operative supplements are not necessary and could be harmful. Anyone who has received steroid therapy within the past 3 months should receive 100 mg hydrocortisone succinate before operation and (following major surgery) the same amount 6-hourly for 3 days to ensure normal plasma corticosteroid levels.

After less severe procedures, treatment for 24 h is sufficient; after minor procedures, 100 mg with premedication is sufficient.


## 7.2  Psychotropic Agents

Monoamine oxidase inhibitors are prescribed for depressive illnesses. Undesirable side-effects arise from inhibition of monoamine oxidase, which inactivates naturally occurring noradrenaline, and certain other enzymes necessary for normal liver function. Liver damage has been reported following its use.

Anaesthesia has two hazards. The first is that of exaggerated response to sympathomimetic drugs, including methylamphetamine, phenylephrine, metaraminol and ephedrine, which all act by increasing the rate of release of noradrenaline from sympathetic nerve terminals. These drugs should therefore be avoided for treatment of hypotensive states.

The second hazardous effect is potentiation of the central depressant action of pethidine, producing signs of overdose, dilated pupils, low blood pressure, depression of respiration and convulsions. The condition responds to intravenous injection of 25 mg hydrocortisone succinate, but if left untreated may be fatal. There is no evidence that opium alkaloids have the same effect. Possibly depression of enzyme activity in the liver by monoamine oxidase inhibitors slows metabolism of pethidine. In spite of the attention given to this hazard, it is difficult to find any authentic published reports of problems occurring in anaesthesia. Two reports which have come to light describe adverse actions when pethidine has been prescribed to relieve acute pain, which presumably resulted in increased adrenergic activity. As these drugs are slowly excreted and 14 days is required for total elimination, it is often not practicable to cease administration before operation. In such cases pethidine is best avoided or alternatively a test dose of 5 mg pethidine could be given intravenously at short intervals until 25 mg has been given. In the absence of adverse reaction it would appear safe to give more if required.

As phenoperidine and fentanyl are derivatives of pethidine they could also have undesirable side-effects in patients receiving monoamine oxidase inhibitors.

The new intravenous agent ketamine (see Sect. 12.3.5) has pronounced sympathetic stimulant properties and should not be administered to patients receiving monoamine oxidase inhibitors.

Tricyclic antidepressants also tend to intensify the action of noradrenaline by preventing reabsorption into the sympathetic nerve cell after release. The main hazard is intensification of the action of adrenaline in local analgesic solutions.

Lithium is of value in the control of manic-depressive psychosis, a form of illness which once under control does not require hospital treatment; hence apparently normal patients may present for anaesthesia who are under lithium treatment. The main hazard of lithium is prolongation of the action of curare and similar muscle relaxants.

## 7.3 Allergy

Drug sensitivity is often confused with allergy. Many patients react adversely to pethidine, for example, complaining of nausea, falling blood pressure and sweating, but no harm results. A repeat prescription is, however, clearly best avoided. This is an example of drug sensitivity.

Allergic reactions occurring in anaesthesia are of two types: anaphylactoid reactions and true anaphylaxis. Anaphylactoid response is more common and follows release of histamine by a drug at the *first* administration. This can happen, for example, with tubocurarine, alphaxalone and alphadolone (see Sect. 12.3.4), certain plasma expanders (Haemaccel) and blood transfusions (see Chap. 21). True anaphylaxis follows repeated administration of a drug which has stimulated antibody formation; at subsequent administrations, histamine release follows formation of antigen-antibody complexes.

Anaphylactic or anaphylactoid reactions can be alarming. They include cardiovascular collapse, bronchospasm and subcutaneous swellings. Treatment is mainly symptomatic: intravenous fluids and vasopressors for cardiovascular collapse and aminophylline and adrenaline for bronchospasm, together with generous doses of hydrocortisone and antihistamine drugs.

# 8 Medicolegal Hazards

## 8.1 Anaesthetists' Responsibilities

As anaesthesia has become more complex, so has the responsibility of those in charge—anaesthetists. The margin of error is much narrower than in any other speciality and lapses which might be unnoticed in another area can result in irreparable damage during anaesthesia or recovery. For this reason, anaesthesia comes at the top of the list of litigation-prone specialities in most defence organisations.

Consultant status implies the capacity to accept total responsibility for all aspects of anaesthesia, whether personally involved or whether the procedure is undertaken by a junior, including pre-operative assessment and recovery as well as the procedure itself. Hazards of assessment are set out in Chaps. 1-7 and it is only necessary to add that a written record of any abnormalities should feature in the patient's record together with an opinion about their significance. It is quite justifiable, and indeed advisable, to call in the assistance of medical colleagues for their opinion, as well as to confer with the surgeon concerned, who must be cognisant of the facts relative to operative and overall risk.

As will be emphasised later, written records are important everywhere, but particularly in the United States, where litigation is commoner and biased in favour of patients. Damages are often astronomical and insurance cover (when obtainable) correspondingly expensive.

The preparation of apparatus and its checking come within the area of responsibility of anaesthetists, although faults arising from defective maintenance of machines or of piped gas supply devolve on the hospital authority or clinic management concerned. The hazards of faulty maintenance, inadequate checking, etc., are considered in greater depth in Chap. 10.

The actual technique employed has recently become of some significance. Failure to ensure unconsciousness is actionable and claims arising from this source are settled out of court every year. It has even been suggested that the agent used could also be the basis of litigation.

Anaesthetic mishaps, when they do occur, arise most often from inexperience and delay in recognising danger signs; others arise from mechanical failure of apparatus; accidents connected with intubation (see Chap. 14) form another important group.

A final consultant responsibility is to ensure adequate anaesthetic records, particularly, as we shall see, when a catastrophe occurs.

## 8.2  Definitions of Negligence

In the public mind, negligence is assumed if patients suffer harm for which the anaesthetist can be held responsible, during an anaesthetic. As already mentioned, the margin for error in anaesthesia is less than in other specialities, and this in itself demands a high standard of performance. Equally, such standards are expected by the law when judgement comes to be pronounced.

However, many cases are not so simple and 'res ipsa loquitur' (the fact speaks for itself) does not always apply. One great judge, Lord Denning, in Hatcher v. Black 1954, has said,

No matter what care was used there was always a *risk* and it would be wrong to say that, simply because a mishap occurred, the hospital and doctors were liable. The jury must not find a doctor negligent simply because a risk inherent in an operation took place or because, in a matter of opinion, he made an error of judgement. They should only find him guilty when he had falled short of the standard of reasonable medical care.

In other words, anaesthetists who do their best for patients insofar as their experience allows, and exercise continuous care and unremitting attention for the entire period of absence of consciousness, stand in little risk of litigation, since accidents in such circumstances are unlikely, and if they were to occur would probably be of a minor nature.

On the other hand, leaving patients in the care of unqualified assistants for a phone call or coffee and reading a newspaper during the procedure are examples of lack of adequate care, and accidents resulting therefrom could be classed as due to negligence.

Another judge, in Maher v. Osborne, talking of a surgoen (but it could just as well apply to an anaesthetist) said,

If he professes an art he must be reasonably skilled in it. He must be careful, but the standard of care which the law requires is not an insurance against accidental slips or accidents . . . it is such a degree of care as normally skilled members of the profession may be reasonably expected to exercise in the actual circumstances of the case in question.

Thus, the status of the person concerned will always receive consideration in assessing the standard of care to be expected. But, also, responsibility can sometimes be shifted to a superior, i.e. a consultant, for permitting a junior to undertake a procedure or accept responsibilities for which adequate training has not been given. There are several instances where this ruling has been involved, especially in anaesthesia.

## 8.3  Procedure Following a Mishap

Whether the mishap was minor, such as an abrasion to lips or damage to a crowned tooth, or major, such as cardiac arrest, fullest records must always be made either at the time or as soon afterwards as possible. One cannot do better than quote Professor Keith Simpson in his first John Snow Memorial Lecture:

> Records are often a serious stumbling block in the path of lawyers who are asked to construct a defence. They are often scrappy enough under peaceful conditions . . . but when there is a crisis in the operating theatre they tend to deteriorate still futher. Such lapses may be understandable but not excusable in the eyes of lawyers. In too many instances, cases quite capable of defence have to be abandoned for lack of vital information about how the accident happened and the steps taken to deal with it.

These criticisms apply especially to Great Britain, where records are notoriously poor and brief, one reason being that turnover is more rapid than in other countries, where the employment of nurse-technicians spreads the work.

Two other points in procedure to be followed after a mishap concern attendance at post-mortems and contact with relatives. In Great Britain an autopsy is compulsory for all patients dying within 24 h of operation. Whether or not the anaesthetic technique is involved, the attendance of the anaesthetist who gave the anaesthetic should be a routine obligation. Anaesthetists and pathologists both benefit. Knowledge of the circumstances is essential for a fair autopsy report, whilst the anaesthetist can acquaint the pathologist with circumstances occurring before or during the procedure which are relevant, and of which the pathologist could not be aware.

The attitude of nursing and medical staff to relatives can be a deciding factor as to whether litigation does or does not take place. If, after a mishap, relatives receive a full and frank explanation and an impression of concern on the part of the anaesthetist, they are often unwilling to proceed. On the other hand, if evasive attempts are made to minimise the mishap or, worse still, contradictory statements are given by different members of the staff, suspicions arise and lead to litigation, often not so much for personal gain as in order to make sure such things do not occur in the future. Professor Simpson emphasises that 'courtesy and a conciliatory approach is more likely to achieve reason and some understanding of the difficulties and the risks involved . . . than hectoring, aggressive behaviour or a shamed silence . . . and that to adopt such an attitude is in no sense an admission of liability.'

## 8.4  Preparation for a Court Case

When a statement of claim has been made, and opinions of experts suggest the defence is reasonable, the defending lawyers will wish to discuss the case with the anaesthetist in order to brief counsel. Some lawyers specialise in this work and are familiar with medical terminology, whilst others may require detailed explanation of what appears trivial to the anaesthetist, who should therefore be prepared to enter into detail about all the circumstances, especially the reasons for undertaking procedures, and if risks were involved, whether any warning was given to relatives.

In the past, a conference with barristers before entering court was considered unethical. Opinions have changed, and counsel prefer to go over a witness's statement, clearing up obscure points and indicating those they desire to emphasise. Many judges feel this avoids misunderstanding and improves the quality of presentation.

## 8.5  Acting as a Medical Witness

Nothing is more vital to success in any legal case than a 'good witness'. This implies a person who can impress a judge or jury with an ability to speak out, give unambiguous answers to questions, and who is never self-contradictory. While some people are naturally good witnesses, others are poor, but all can improve their performance by attending to certain fundamental rules.

Knowledge of all the facts of the case, and the tactics counsel intend to pursue, is indispensable. This involves detailed study of statements and thought about the personal evidence and where it would come under attack in cross-examination.

Conduct in the witness box is very important. Doctors in the witness box are often apt to forget that lay people, barristers and judges especially, do not understand medical jargon. The use of simple descriptive terms is essential at all times. For example, to say 'type of breathing' is preferable to saying 'pattern of respiration', 'heart beat' is preferable to 'cardiac rhythm'. On the other hand, over-simplification and an attitude of condescension can also create a bad impression. One cannot stress too strongly also the need not to give views on unfamiliar specialities or matters and to have no fear of expressing ignorance on matters outside one's special field of knowledge. Often counsel will, for reasons of their own, tempt witnesses to make statements which could subsequently be used against them.

Cross-examination is inevitable and witnesses should prepare themselves both mentally and emotionally. Great concentration is vital, and a pause to assemble thoughts before answering completely justifiable. Emotions should play no part and, as it were, be kept on ice, for often counsel can be provoking. Firmness must not be confused with inflexibility, and if a view is questioned, one can reasonably claim that one's view is that 'generally accepted' or that 'of many of my colleagues' rather than persist that it is a universal view.

Finally, as a help to witnesses, Professor Simpson has drawn up a list of 'bias words' by which counsel endeavour to use expressions more to their advantage and rather destructive of the medical witnesses.

| Where the expert has used: | Counsel may suggest: |
| --- | --- |
| Opinion | Guesswork |
| View | Conjecture |
| Belief | Theory |
| Convinced | Prejudiced |
| Co-operation | Collusion |
| Logical | Plausible |
| Self-evident | Meretricious or glib |
| Current view | Present-day theory |

When counsel attempts to change words in this way, witness is entitled to correct him, interrupting if necessary, and protesting against misquotation by saying, 'I do not recollect using that word', or some such phrase. Medical witnesses usually receive considerate treatment from courts but they should not depend on it and be ready to make preparations for appearance just as seriously as they do for the anaesthetics which they undertake every day.

# 9 Occupational Hazards

Written record of concern for the health of persons working in operating theatres dates back to a paper published in 1929 by the Institute of Hygiene, Berlin, where, 10 years earlier, mechanical means of removing anaesthetic vapours from operating theatres had been installed. The paper considered that anaesthetic vapours were potentially harmful, and that environmental factors such as standing, humidity, and poor illumination also contributed. Although no scientific evidence for toxicity was available in animal experiments, the Institute recommended immediate action to remove anaesthetic vapours from operating suites since it felt it would be unwise to wait for conclusive evidence.

There has been little change in the position since that time, in spite of the appearance during the past 10 years of over 200 papers on this subject. Although absolute proof of harm is lacking, most hospital administrations consider (like the Germans) that to wait for proof would not be sensible and the expense of the institution of some preventive measures is justified. This has encouraged the assumption in some quarters that atmospheric pollution is a proven hazard, which in its turn leads to the assumption that unexplained malaise, aches or pains arising during employment in operating suites were caused by pollution. The best way of dispelling such alarmist attitudes is to make a brief dispassionate review of some of the evidence available. This divides itself into the hazards affecting reproduction, i.e. miscarriages and congenital malformations in infants (teratogenicity), hazards affecting general health, and hazards affecting professional performance, i.e. fatigue, stress and tedium.

## 9.1 Hazards Affecting Reproduction

### 9.1.1 Miscarriage

In 1967 a paper appeared in Russia drawing attention to a possible increase in the incidence of miscarriages amongst female staff in operating theatres. Although the enquiry was aimed at an assessment of general working conditions, it revealed a surprising miscarriage rate of 58%, the normal average being about 25%. In this survey, which comprised 354 doctors, only 110 were women and of these only 31 were pregnant and thus the subjects of the detailed survey. They were aged between 24 and 28 years, and 18 miscarried. There were no controls nor is there any information about how the questionnaire was conducted. Most authorities regard these figures with some reservation and feel there must be other circumstances involved.

The Russian paper evoked much interest and encouraged other surveys. A report from Denmark showed that, although there was an increase in miscarriages amongst nurse anaesthetists and female medical anaesthetists, a similar increase was also apparent in unexposed wives of anaesthetists.

Two further investigations, one in the United States and one in Finland, were conducted with nurses as well as anaesthetists. In the United States, nurses working in operating rooms and general duty nurses were interviewed at length by a nurse and a psychologist. Fifty anaesthetists and 81 physicians were interrogated through a detailed questionnaire sent by mail. The Finnish series included 124 theatre nurses, 43 intensive care nurses, 53 anaesthetists and 75 casualty nurses. Both series showed a small but statistically significant increase in the overall miscarriage rate but both included, as noted, operating room nurses and nurse anaesthetists. The response rate in both series was only 70% and if one considers that those with positive information are more likely to take the trouble to report than those without, the 30% failure could include many negative returns and possibly tip the statistical scales towards non-significance.

A British questionnaire by mail which included controls and had an 80% response rate confirmed a very slight (1.24:1) but statistically significant increase in frequency of miscarriage amongst anaesthetists, with no difference whether they were working or not during pregnancy. Slight increase in minor congenital abnormalities was noted.

The American Society of Anaesthetists carried out a large-scale investigation whose title, 'Committee on the Effect of Trace Anaesthetics on the Health of Operating Room Personnel' has been criticised because 'it unscientifically prejudges the answer to the question.' This survey also confirmed an increased risk of spontaneous miscarriage amongst women working in operating rooms but it offered no support to the possibility of male exposure resulting in the wife miscarrying, as had been suggested by the Danish survey.

*Comment.* A statistical increase in the incidence of miscarriages in operating theatre personnel (but not anaesthetists) is apparent from surveys carried out in widely scattered countries. This has resulted in recommendations in Great Britain, the United States and Canada for the installation of systems for removal of anaesthetic vapours from operating rooms known as scavenging systems. However, the authorities are careful to give no recommendations for minimal figures of concentration, nor for the maximum time of exposure. These recommendations are, of course, measures of prudence, and are not based on any evidence that anaesthetic vapours are the cause. The following considerations suggest that other factors must be involved:

1) If anaesthetic vapours were the cause one would expect a higher rate of miscarriage to occur in those with greatest exposure, but there is no difference of incidence between operating room staff with minimal exposure and anaesthetists and anaesthetic nurses with maximum exposure. Published statistics show that incidence of miscarriage reported amongst operating staff is higher in the United States than in the United Kingdom. This, despite the fact that routine use of carbon dioxide absorption and low flow rates plus air conditioning in the United States, surely results in lower average atmospheric contamination than in the United Kingdom, where high flow rates are commonplace, air conditioning is rarely found and in many instances the ventilation is rather defective.

2) If anaesthetic vapours were the reason for miscarriages, then removal from exposure should lower the rate.

The A.S.A. survey showed that vacation for a year or more prior to pregnancy did not alter the miscarriage rate in nurses or MD anaesthetists. In addition, operating room nurses and technicians not exposed to vapours in the operating room during pregnancy had a rate lower than operating room nurses and technicians who were exposed, but equal to the control. Taken with the figures above for those leaving the operating room for a year, this is surely convincing evidence that the hazard in question is certainly not concerned with anaesthetic vapours.

3) Exposure of animals to operating theatre concentrations for seven to eight hours, five days a week, throughout pregnancy had no adverse effects on reproduction (see Sect. 9.1.3).

4) Women are widely employed in the dry-cleaning industry where they are exposed to quite appreciable concentrations of commercial trichloroethylene containing impurities. If anaesthetic vapour were conducive to miscarriages, or liver disease, here are the ideal conditions, yet industrial medical literature contains no reference to these complaints. The only ill effects appear to be headache, lassitude and nausea.

### 9.1.2 Congenital Abnormalities

The statistical standards for significance used in the A.S.A. group have been criticised, especially in respect of the incidence of congenital abnormalities. If 5% had been used as the level of significance, neither the women in the A.S.A., nor those in the operating room nurse and technician group had children with a significantly higher rate of abnormalities than the control, nor did absence from the operating room for one year reduce the incidence.

### 9.1.3  Animal Experimentation

There have been several studies on the effects of trace anaesthetics on reproduction in animals. Halothane at 16 parts per million, equivalent to the concentration found in operating theatres, given seven hours a day, five days a week for six weeks had no effect on reproduction in rats, although the reverse held good for similar exposure to nitrous oxide at one thousand parts per million. A further study increasing the concentration of halothane to one hundred parts per million had no effect on the rats.

A study involving administration of halothane at the high concentration of five hundred parts per million to young female rats throughout pregnancy had no effect on reproductive abilities compared with controls breathing pure air. These findings must surely dispel any lingering doubts that halothane is a factor in the occurrence of miscarriage in operating room personnel.

Much of the data which shows an increase in teratogenicity arises from exposure of animals to between one hundred and one thousand times the concentration found in operating theatres and hence is irrelevant in the clinical context. The animal work quoted above on pregnant rats was negative with respect to teratogenicity. The subject, however, is one of great complexity because animal susceptibility varies widely. In mice, for example, one day's isolation and deprivation of food on the fifteenth day of pregnancy is sufficient to induce development of a cleft palate.

## 9.2  General Health Hazards

The A.S.A. study included questionnaires to cover the incidence of neoplasms and liver and kidney disease amongst anaesthetists. The questionnaire could be criticised for generating bias, since the section dealing with health had the following headings: Liver ? Kidney ? Other ? More recently, a study has been undertaken in Glasgow on the same subject.

### 9.2.1  A.S.A. Study

*Neoplasms.* The A.S.A. study showed no differences between male anaesthetists and controls. Had a 1% level of significance been used, no difference between female anaesthetists doctors and operating theatre nurses and their controls would have been seen either.

Nurse anaesthetists showed an increase in cancer rate compared with controls, but critics point out that these figures include some findings from Michigan, where the rate was found to be twice that of the controls. The nurses in Michigan were surveyed twice and thus subject to sampling bias. A recalculation omitting these nurses might give a more reliable figure.

*Liver Disease*. The A.S.A. reported a higher incidence of liver disease (excluding serum hepatitis) amongst women working in operating theatres than in the controls. The questionnaire specifically excluded serum hepatitis as a cause of liver disease, because this is known to be more frequent amongst operating theatre staff. However, in the form the nurses were asked to fill in, the space for diagnosis of liver disease did not include sufficient information to separate the varieties. It is suggested that many of those who entered 'hepatitis' forgot that they had only contracted serum hepatitis. Even so, amongst male nurse anaesthetists there was no significant difference with the controls, and had the 1% level of significanc been used for female anaesthetists, there would have been no difference with them either.

*Kidney Disease*. Results concerning kidney disease were contradictory. No evidence appeared that male anaesthetists were more prone to kidney disease than the controls (indeed the paediatricians had a higher incidence) nor was the overall rate for females different. At a 1% level of significance, there was some difference between nurse anaesthetists and their controls but no indication exists of the type of disease (although pyelonephritis and pyelitis were said to be excluded).

### 9.2.2 Glasgow Study

The information from the Glasgow study is not yet fully collated. Preliminary findings suggest that an illness is more frequently reported amongst anaesthetists than in the control groups. There also appears to be a raised incidence of peptic ulcer and cardiovascular disease. There does not, however, seem to be any difference of incidence of neoplasms between anaesthetists, doctors and the lay public.

### 9.3 Anaesthetists' Professional Performance

In some respects it is a pity that incidence of miscarriage and attempts to relate it to trace concentrations of anaesthetic vapours have drawn attention away from more immediate problems concerning the effects of work load and the nature and duration of operations, upon individual performance and overall safety. These are items themselves that could have more relation to the incidence of miscarriage than the inhalation of low concentrations of anaesthetic vapours.

All kinds of test have been devised to determine the effect of prolonged inhalation of low concentrations of anaesthetic vapours as found in operating theatres and around the patient's expiratory valve. They, no doubt, contribute to the overall feelings of lassitude and fatigue which many experience during and at the conclusion of long and tedious operations.

One writer defined anaesthesia as ninety-nine per cent boredom and one per cent panic. Others have compared it to the aircraft pilot's task, where take-off and landing correspond to induction and recovery, and the period in flight with the automatic pilot is compared to maintenance with relaxant and mechanical ventilator. These comparisons over-simplify the problem.

A well-conducted anaesthetic requires a level of concentration unequalled in any other branch of medicine (including surgery) in order to detect, interpret at any one moment and, if necessary, correct small changes in the physiological state of the patient. For a surgeon, an operation is, more often than not, a repetitive technical exercise whose possible difficulties are well known beforehand, as are the standard ways of overcoming them. A surgeon's anxieties arise in the pre-operative phase, in the making of a diagnosis and the decision when and how to operate, and during the postoperative phase. For these reasons, surgeons can continue to operate happily all day sustained by occasional pauses for solid and liquid food and finish not unduly fatigued, whilst their anaesthetic colleague is reduced to a limp, mentally exhausted person who can hardly raise concentration sufficiently to read the headlines of a newspaper.

The reasons for this mental exhaustion lie in the constant observations which anaesthetists must make in the course of any general anaesthetic. Some idea of the detail involved can be obtained from consideration of the information that is constantly entering the central nervous system of anaesthetists through their eyes, ears and hands.

*Eyes.* The eyes make the following observations:

1) Skin: cyanotic or pink, indicating respiratory inadequacy or other-wise; or pale and sweaty suggesting haemorrhage or shock.

2) Head and neck: movements of the eyes indicating light anaes-thesia. State of the pupil—dilated after atropine, but can indicate deep anaesthesia, a ganglion blocker, acute oxygen lack and/or respiratory and cardiac failure.

3) Chest: movement of the chest—is air entering the lungs and expansion equal on both sides? If the patient is breathing spontaneously the nature of respiratory rhythm changes with varying depth. A tracheal tug indicates inadequate reversal of relaxants whilst retraction of the intercostal muscles in the lower part of the chest indicates respiratory obstruction.

4) Abdomen: during laparotomy, observation of the surgical man-ipulations, judging whether relaxation is adequate, or is the patient

straining? Is haemorrhage excessive? How much blood is going into the sucker? How much soiling is there of the peritoneum? (This has relation to postoperative shock.)

5) Apparatus: Do the rotameters show adequate gas flow? Are the contents of the cylinders adequate? Are the vaporiser settings right? Is there anaesthetic in the vaporiser? Does the pop-off valve need adjusting? Does the bag fill adequately? If soda lime is in use, what is the colour? Is it exhausted? Check the ventilator settings: inflation pressures, rate of inflation, the presence or absence of negative pressure. Does the ventilator fill the chest? Is it connected properly? Are the flow rates adequate? Check the amount and the rate of intravenous infusion; if blood is used, check the bottle numbers and the patient's number. Make sure the blood is correct for that patient.

6) Physiological measurements: the pulse and blood pressure must be taken and recorded every five minutes; likewise the readings of the cardiac monitor if in use, or the flashing light of a pulse monitor. The blood loss record must be noted throughout the operation.

7) Is the operation progressing according to plan or is there a change? What extra difficulties face the surgeon? Is the blood loss excessive? If a tourniquet applied, is the pressure adequate?

*Ears.* Anaesthetists use their ears almost unconsciously during an operation. Listening to the exhalations through the expiratory valve, even small changes can rapidly be picked up; also any change in the noise made by the ventilator and its rhythm is immediately detected. Airline pilots develop the same facility and note any change in rhythm or pitch of their engines very quickly even though engaged in conversation. Stethoscopes are often used during anaesthesia, a precordial stethoscope is essential to monitor the respiration and heart rate of children, as well as for recording blood pressure. The nature of spontaneous respiration offers information, laryngospasm suggests light anaesthesia: a pause after expiration indicates a light plane of anaesthesia and a pause after inspiration indicates a deeper plane of anaesthesia with relaxation of abdominal muscles. Cardiac and pulse monitors can deliver audible signals which are disturbed by diathermy or other electrical equipment and cease suddenly if someone trips over the lead wire.

Ears also have to endure 'noises off' and irrelevant conversation. Such noises can distract concentration and cause irritation. Anaesthetists have the right to insist on silence even if it means workmen ceasing their activities. Some surgeons enjoy piped music. It should never be played in an anaesthetic room during induction.

Silence in the anaesthetic room should be the rule and conversation strictly prohibited. Even whispers can become audible to a patient at a certain stage of induction. During surgery only the surgeon and anaesthetist may initiate conversation. Anaesthetists should take care not to disturb the surgeon with conversation when he is at a delicate part of the operation. However, during long and tedious operations, a pause for small talk at intervals—even the cracking of a feeble joke—provides some mental relaxation and temporary relief from continued concentration.

*Hands.* A finger on the pulse is worth several monitors. It gives an indication of pulse rate and the presence or otherwise of cardiac arrhythmias. It helps to maintain contact between anaesthetists and their patients. The feel of the skin is important: dry warm skin indicates a good clinical state, cold and clammy indicates operative shock. By pressure or friction of the skin one can gain an indication of the adequacy of perfusion by noting the capillary refill time.

# Part II

*Considerations Relevant to*
*All Procedures*

# 10 Preparation and Use of Anaesthetic Apparatus

## 10.1  General Remarks

Some form of anaesthetic apparatus is indispensable for the conduct of modern anaesthesia. Although designs vary in each country and between countries, there are basic functions common to all, and all carry similar hazards, particularly when used without proper care.

The following are common to all anaesthetic machines and all carry some degree of hazard:

1) Source of gases—cylinders or centralised pipelines

2) Flowmeters to measure the gas flow to the patient

3) Vaporisers for liquid anaesthetics

4) Rebreathing or reservoir bags with corrugated tubing to bring gases and vapours to the patient

5) Arrangements and responsibility for regular maintenance

Probably the greatest hazard is an unfamiliar apparatus, and it constitutes the greatest folly to start an anaesthetic on an unfamiliar and unchecked machine. Apart from routine checks before use of any machine (which the contents of this chapter should make obvious), anyone using an unfamiliar machine must make sure of (a) the position of the emergency oxygen supply and its being in working order; (b) the arrangement of the flowmeters and the source of gas supply, whether piped or cylinder; (c) the type and calibration of vaporisers, together with any relevant scales and slide-rules required to check the concentration; (d) the presence or absence of dual gas circuits—one for an absorber and an alternative one for direct high flow methods. Failure to recognise these can result in embarrassing attempts to anaesthetise with air and (when a ventilator is included in the absorber circuit) progressive hypoxia, which is difficult to detect clinically in the early stages.

In most modern theatre suites with piped gases, there are often two anaesthetic machines, one for induction of anaesthesia in the anaesthetic room and the other for maintenance in the theatre. These machines may not always be of the same design nor is the machine in the theatre always connected up to the pipe supply, and it is the responsibility of anaesthetists to make sure that the second machine is checked over, as well as the one in the anaesthetic room, before starting to induce anaesthesia.

Nobody should be ashamed to admit ignorance about unfamiliar apparatus or to ask advice from a local nurse or technician who assembles and maintains the equipment.

## 10.2 Gas Supply

Gas supply for anaesthetic apparatus is either from cylinders attached to the machine or from a central piped supply. Both sources of supply carry their own particular risks. Lack of uniformity in this respect of itself constitutes a hazard, since someone accustomed, for example, to central piped supply who then goes to work in an area dependent on cylinders may (having got out of the habit) fail to check the content of the oxygen cylinder.

### 10.2.1 Piped Gases

When first introduced into anaesthetic practice, piped gases were claimed to offer added protection against accidental failure of supplies. But experience has shown that accidents can still happen.

Cross-connection of oxygen and nitrous oxide pipelines during construction has been responsible for as many as 44 fatalities in Canada and the United States, but in the United Kingdom a detailed procedure for testing newly installed pipelines before acceptance from contractors should avoid such catastrophes.

Cross-connection between hoses carrying gases from gas outlets to anaesthetic machines has been the source of two serious accidents (one fatal) and measures have been introduced to prevent their repetition.

In the early days of piped supplies old machines were adapted by placing a 'Schrader' type valve onto the old cylinder blocks into which a spigot attached to the supply tubing could be plugged and removed quickly, should it be necessary. Although the hoses were clearly colour coded, the probes were interchangeable—an unsafe arrangement. In addition the supply hoses were manufactured in three different diameters and each required a matching spigot. Inevitably at some time, the wrong size of spigot (too small) found its way onto the gas tubing, so that a loose joint resulted, which could be separated. If this happened to both oxygen and nitrous oxide on the same apparatus, a sudden strain could result in disconnection of both. Cross-connection could easily be made in the hurry of re-connection and apparently has happened.

To prevent such accidents regulations have been made for the assembly and connection of hoses to gas outlets and anaesthetic machines. The use of the 'Schrader' type valve is no longer allowed. The probe connecting supply tubing to the anaesthetic apparatus must be non-interchangeable and clamped firmly to the tubing by a metal ferrule. Its connection to the anaesthetic apparatus is by a threaded connection, screwed securely by a spanner, preferably to a point separate from the old cylinder blocks. The probe joining the piped gas outlet to the tubing is also non-interchangeable and firmly joined to the pressure tubing by a metal ferrule, so that disconnection is almost impossible.

There are several checking procedures for new machines or machines newly connected to pipelines. The chief objectives are to ensure that only one flowmeter operates when the appropriate control tap is opened, thus excluding the possibility of interconnection. Pressure tests are also undertaken to exclude leaks.

*'Permit to Work' System.* The words 'permit to work' are rather misleading. The system is not a way of overcoming a 'closed shop' or lines of demarcation, but an attempt to ensure safety during and after servicing, repairing, alteration or extension of piped gas systems. In the past, accidents have happened because well-meaning unqualified staff have tried to restore interrupted supplies. Difficulties can also arise when the engineering departments or outside contractors interrupt gas supplies without previously informing those who use them.

Maintenance of repairs to pipeline systems involve grades of hospital staff, some of whom may meet for the first time during work on a pipeline. Good co-operation and communication between departments is essential if the work is to proceed smoothly. Work may only begin when it is certain all persons concerned by disturbance of a pipeline know the date, time and duration of the interruption (which should not normally be more than 24 h). Medical and nursing staff working in the area, the pharmacy, specialised contractors and various grades of engineering staff all need to be informed. Until this is assured the hospital administration should not approve a permit to work. Permits to work are not of course necessary for replacement of cylinders and recharging with liquid oxygen, provided no disturbance of the service is involved.

The permit to work system recognises three degrees of hazards of work on pipelines: high, medium and low.

*High* hazard arises when there is disturbance of in-service pipelines involving a risk of cross-connection and/or of atmospheric pollution.

*Medium* hazards include work on terminal units with more than one medical gas (as in most anaesthetic departments). A hazard of cross-connection does exist, but it will become minimal when hoses are fitted with non-interchangeable connections and the probes to the anaesthetic apparatus are secured to the hose by screwed and ferruled connections.

*Low* hazard includes work on terminal units if there is a piped source of only one gas and if the terminal complies with British standards. Work on some older terminals which do not incorporate an integral isolating valve (BOC Mark I and II and Draeger old pattern) can entail cutting off supplies to a complete ward or department, with whom the closest co-operation is necessary, as well as a permit to work.

For further details of the permit to work system, the Department of Health and Social Security's guidelines should be consulted (see Selective Bibliography).

### 10.2.2  Cylinder Gases

Cylinder identification and connection to machines still constitute a hazard, although in Great Britain and Ireland colour coding and pin index systems are uniform and satisfactory. Until this system gains international acceptance, those who travel abroad should be on their guard and take care to check local cylinder colour customs and whether pin index systems are in use. In the United States there have recently been recommendations to bring the cylinder coding into line with Great Britain's.

Although satisfied that cylinders contain what they appear to contain, an anaesthetist is still in ignorance about how much they contain and how long they may be used before they become empty. Most oxygen-reducing valves incorporate a pressure gauge, which unfortunately is not always accurate. Again, in unfamiliar surroundings, someone in the theatre area may know if a dial is faulty but may not volunteer the information unless asked. A recent hazard arose when a non-return valve on a cylinder attachment yoke became stuck, cutting off supply of oxygen from one cylinder, although the dial registered 'full'. This apparatus, although it originally was constructed for cylinder use with pressures up to 13 600 kPa, was changed to a pipeline with a much lower pressure (410 kPa)—insufficient to open the non-return valve, so no gas flowed. Steps have now been taken to replace the existing valve on this machine with one of a new design.

Anaesthetists in general should decline to start an anaesthetic with an oxygen cylinder registering less than 350 kPa and to change cylinders during an anaesthetic as soon as pressure reaches this level. If this is not done and, as has happened in the past, the anaesthetist's attention is momentarily diverted by an emergency arising at the surgical end (e.g. from haemorrhage), it is quite easy for the cylinder to run out whilst the anaesthetist is paying attention to the intravenous infusion.

### 10.2.3 Oxygen Failure Indicators

Oxygen failure has such devastating consequences that anaesthetists would be justified in insisting that every apparatus carries an effective failure-warning device that should be tested and certified every day the machine is used. There are anaesthetists who pride themselves on their vigilance and constant observation, confident that they can always detect oxygen lack before any harm takes place. No doubt such supermen exist, but the average patient is in the hands of the average anaesthetist in whom fatigue, monotony, and preoccupation with infusions, operative haemorrhage, or faulty monitors may all contribute to failure to notice the decline of an oxygen flowmeter to the zero point. In Great Britain and Ireland, two types of failure-warning devices are in use, although one, the Bosun, is no longer produced.

The Bosun gives warning of oxygen failure either by a red light operated by a battery or by a whistle operated by a nitrous oxide cylinder. The apparatus was never 100% reliable because often there was no battery in the battery holder or the battery had been left in the holder too long and had seized up and was impossible to move. Moreover, there is an on/off switch on the machine, and if this happens to be turned to 'off', the whistle does not operate.

The most recent warning device announces oxygen failure with a low-pitched wolf-whistle, unmistakable and certain to attract attention. At the same time, the nitrous oxide supply is cut off, so that all that is left for the patient to breathe is air which can be entrained into the circuit.

Another device, known as the Quantiflex M.D. Mixer, allows dialling of any oxygen percentage from 30% to 100%. The nitrous oxide automatically closes if the oxygen supply falls below the set level.

The only sure way of detecting oxygen lack in an anaesthetic circuit is to include a reliable oxygen concentration meter in the breathing system. Although that would be ideal, it is too expensive to bring into general use.

## 10.3 Rotameters

The position of oxygen rotameters at the left, i.e. the upstream position, is hazardous. If a crack occurs in the glass tube carrying either the oxygen, or cyclopropane or nitrous oxide, oxygen will leak through in sufficient quantity to cause hypoxia. If the oxygen rotameter is placed at the extreme right or downstream position of the rotameter block, none of these dangerous situations can arise. Anaesthetists in the United States have agreed that in future all new equipment should have the rotameter in this position. It is admitted that this change could give rise to mistakes of 'touch' identification. To avoid this the oxygen control knob in the new position is to be fitted with characteristic projections making identification quite simple, whilst all other flow control knobs will be made smooth and round as at present. British manufacturers have overcome this disadvantage by retaining the oxygen flowmeter in its original position but directing the oxygen flow through a by-pass which joins the other gases in the downstream position. Dangers can also arise from loose controls of the rotameters or their inadvertent turning on or off during a tense moment in induction or intubation. A loose oxygen control can easily be closed by an observer's sleeve rubbing against it, especially if the bank of flowmeters is prominent and sticks out as it does in some mechanical ventilators. This is another reason for placing the oxygen in the downstream position.

Inadvertent opening of flowmeters can easily escape notice if the bobbin becomes jammed at the top of the tube. This is particularly likely to happen with cyclopropane, because the flowmeter bobbin is very small and its disappearance can easily escape notice. For this reason it is better to keep the cyclopropane cylinder itself closed rather than to depend on the fine control of the rotameter.

## 10.4  Vaporisers

### 10.4.1  Copper Kettle

The copper kettle vaporiser is popular in the United States for its versatility. It can be used for any volatile agent, because the amount of vapour delivered can be calculated from the gas flow, the ambient temperature and the vaporisation coefficient of the anaesthetic. There are, however, practical hazards. Old models filled from the top and without any indication of the maximum filling level, so that over-filling and delivery of liquid anaesthetic to the breathing circuit could occur with potentially fatal results. The new copper kettles have the filling port on the side at the maximum safe level, making over-filling impossible.

There is nothing to prevent mixing two different agents in a copper kettle. This is more likely if several anaesthetists use the same machine. A fatality has been recorded from this cause following anaesthesia with a mixture of trichloroethylene and halothane through a closed circuit. This error could be prevented by fitting a detachable specific filling and emptying device which, unfortunately, is not at present available. Anaesthetists should always empty a copper kettle after use as well as examining its interior for contents before adding any agent at the start of an anaesthesia.

### 10.4.2 Temperature Compensated Vaporisers

The Fluotec, Tritec and Pentec deliver selected concentrations of halothane, trichloroethylene and methoxyflurane, irrespective of the ambient temperature. They do, however, require annual checking for accuracy. When more than one vaporiser is placed on an anaesthetic apparatus, connection is usually in series and carries potential danger. If accidentally a second vaporiser is left open and contains anaesthetic, a mixture of anaesthetics can be received by the patient. Incorrect filling is a hazard. Should rapidly vaporising halothane be put into a Pentec designed for slow vaporising methoxyflurane, patients could receive up to 8% halothane, possibly with fatal results. Errors in filling can be avoided by a pin index safety filler system; such systems are now available in the United Kingdom and the United States. Alternatively, as with the copper kettle, every vaporiser should be emptied after use and only filled by an anaesthetist.

### 10.4.3 Glass Vaporisers

Two forms commonly found on anaesthetic apparatus that are not temperature compensated are the Boyle's bottle and the smaller, Goldman vaporiser. It is rare at the present time for a large Boyle's bottle to be used for any agent other than trichloroethylene. The use of a large Boyle's bottle for halothane is potentially dangerous because it is almost impossible to control in any reasonable way the percentage of halothane which it will deliver. The reason for this is that the controls on these bottles are designed for use with ether, and ether requires a large volume of gas flow in order to achieve the high percentage of 20% or 25% required to induce anaesthesia. These large bottles were used in the early days of halothane. They delivered unnecessarily large percentages, which may account for some of the reports of overdosage and certainly for reports of increased vaginal bleeding in gynaecological and obstetric operations when halothane was first introduced.

Boyle's vaporisers should never be used for administration of halothane. If a temperature compensated vaporiser is not available a small compact vaporiser, the Goldman, should be used since the maximum concentration obtainable does not exceed 2%.

### 10.4.4 Possible Back-Pressure Effect

It has been suggested that with a low flow of gases and artificial ventilation, a rise in back pressure in the circuit during the inspiratory phase is sometimes transmitted to the vaporiser, thus increasing the production of vapour. Reports on this possibility are contradictory and appear to depend on the type of vaporiser; indeed, falls in concentration have been reported with a Fluotec used with some ventilators (namely the Blease and the Barnett).

### 10.4.5  Conclusion

At all times and especially before using a strange machine, a check on vaporisers should be made before use to ensure that controls are in the 'off' position and that they contain the correct fluids. If more than one vaporiser is included in the circuit, it should be a rule that all are emptied at the end of the working day. The following day the anaesthetist who is to use that machine should fill the vaporisers personally and thus be responsible for their contents.


## 10.5  Breathing Circuits

### 10.5.1  Hose Connections

In recent years, all hose connections in the United Kingdom and Ireland have been made to conform to British Standards, i.e. male plug into female socket on all connections between the apparatus and the patient and, when a circuit is in use, between the patient and the apparatus. That is to say, the same fittings pass in the same direction in a circle. Unfortunately, the early plastic models were very unstable, and it was not an unusual experience, following an intravenous induction, when one picked up the breathing attachments, to have the whole assembly fall to pieces on the floor. Frequent experience of this demoralising accident provoked one humorist to call out in a loud voice whenever it happened, 'British Standards strike again!' One reason for this periodic collapse is said to be the accumulation of grease and lubricant on the connections. Periodic cleaning with a grease-solvent such as trichloroethylene increases their security considerably. Substitution of metal for plastic has brought about some improvement, but a clip-on connection which cannot fall apart still needs to be designed. This is especially important when the hoses are hidden under towels (drapes), since it is not always possible to see if they become detached.

When two circuits, a high-flow and a low-flow circle absorber circuit, exist on the same machine, the gas supply plug may have to be changed when one converts from one to the other. Unless this is checked before use, a patient can be connected to a circuit which is providing neither oxygen nor anaesthetic.

### 10.5.2  Obstruction and Increased Airway Pressure

Over-inflation of lungs by anaesthetic gases is by no means rare and some anaesthetists maintain it has been responsible for surgical deaths previously ascribed to other causes. Obstruction to outflow of gases when fresh gases continue to enter the circuit can result in a build-up of pressure in any of the following ways:

1) Failure to open the Heidbrink or 'pop-off' valve
2) Accidental failure to include the Heidbrink valve in the circuit

3) Kinking the outlet tube of an Ayre's T-piece circuit

4) Locking a Ruben valve in the 'inspiratory' position, thus closing the expiratory port, more likely to happen when total flow of gases exceeds the minute volume

In all these circumstances, the presence of a *rubber* reservoir bag in circuit confers a degree of protection to the patient. Pressure in rubber bags seldom exceeds 8 kPa. Laplace's law $P = T/R$ applies. Elasticity of the bag allows considerable expansion in circumstances in which the ratio between the elastic tension $T$ and the radius $R$ remains constant, thus pressure does not increase. When the limit of elasticity is reached, elastic tension also reaches its limit and even a small increase in pressure results in a blow-out, so avoiding damage to the patient's lungs.

*Plastic* bags on the other hand lack this protection as no increase in radius is possible; tension remains constant and very high pressures can occur, up to 20 kPa, causing severe damage to the lungs before a blow-out occurs.

Exclusion of rubber reservoir bags from the circuit can occur accidentally, e.g. by omitting to fit the bag, closing it with a tap (old models), misconnecting when a ventilator is in use, incorrect setting of unidirectional valves, or simple kinking of expiratory tubing (more likely if perished). When this happens with conventional gas flows, patients become cyanosed and the anaesthetist, assuming there is a leak in the circuit, is likely to flush the system with the emergency oxygen supply, making matters worse.

When conventional gas flows produce cyanosis, it is far better to dismantle the circuit and test the patency of the airway or tube rather than flush the system with oxygen. Adoption of this rule would avoid fatalities that occur every year from kinked or misplaced endotracheal tubes.

Results of excessive airway pressure depend partly on the manner of its application (moderate or sustained) and partly on the cardiovascular and respiratory status of the patient. Moderate sustained pressure reduces cardiac output more by interference with return of blood from the lungs to the heart than with the venous return from the systemic circulation. Under light general anaesthesia, some compensatory reflex sympathetic vasoconstriction occurs but becomes less effective as anaesthesia deepens or if the patient has received central or peripheral anti-adrenolytic drugs. Sustained moderate pressure is not likely to cause alveolar rupture except in sufferers from emphysema, in whom unilateral pneumothorax may easily occur.

Sudden application of greater pressures, however, ruptures alveoli. Escaped gases enter the pulmonary interstitial tissue and track into the lung hilum along the vascular sheaths, gaining access to the mediastinum and compressing the heart and great vessels; from there they track downwards to produce pneumoperitoneum and upwards to appear as subcutaneous emphysema in the neck. By such time, patients are usually pulseless from a combination of pressure on pulmonary vessels, reduced venous return and cardiac tamponade. Ultimately gas bubbles enter the pulmonary circulation, track back to the heart and produce air embolus, ventricular fibrillation and cardiac arrest. Thus sudden unexpected appearance of subcutaneous emphysema is a sign to detach the apparatus and relieve thoracic and abdominal pressure, either by surgical incision or use of a trocar and cannula or a large aspirating needle.

Such accidents could be prevented by insisting that all breathing circuits carry means of limiting pressure. All modern British apparatus carries a pressure relief valve which protects both the rotameters and the patients by blowing off at 6 kPa. This valve is not adequate for use with certain types of gas-driven ventilators which require a pressure of something like 35 kPa. It has therefore been suggested that all breathing attachments, as distinct from the anaesthetic machine, should carry a pressure limiting valve which goes off at about 4 kPa. Various types are available. One consists of a pressure relief flap valve in rebreathing bags and the others are spring-loaded or dead weight valves which can be installed at some convenient point in the breathing circuit.

### 10.5.3  Leaks in Coaxial Circuits

Concern about atmospheric contamination by anaesthetics has led to modification of methods of gas delivery in order to facilitate disposal of the exhaled gases by scavenging devices. One of these modifications is known as the coaxial circuit. The fresh gases are delivered to the distal end of the Magill or Mapelson corrugated delivery hose by a small-bore flexible inner tube connected to the gas outlet by a rubber sleeve and similarly to the delivery port at the face piece. When the patient exhales, the gases pass out through the wide-bore tube to an expiratory valve placed near the rebreathing bag, from where the waste gases are led away by corrugated tubing to the appropriate scavenging device. In certain models of coaxial circuits, the rubber sleeve at the fresh gas delivery end became torn so that fresh gases entered the large-bore tubing near the expiratory valve and so passed through the expiratory valve when the patient expired, the remainder of the circuit then acting as 'dead space'. Steps have been taken by the manufacturers to prevent this accident occurring again. The transparency of the outer tubing is a help in assessing the continuity of the inner tube but it has been suggested that the manufacturers might design an alternative by placing the fresh gas tubing of small diameter along the outside of the larger tube.

A simple but useful test for leaks in coaxial circuits has been described by Foex and Crampton Smith, and consists of occluding the distal or patient end of the coaxial circuit, either with a finger or the plunger of a 2-cc syringe, with the gases flowing. If, when the circuit is occluded, the rotameters descend slightly, recovering to their original position on removal of the finger, the integrity of the circuit is established. A similar manoeuvre is also a test for a leaking rotameter tube.

### 10.5.4  Other Leaks

In addition to coaxial circuits, the average circle carbon dioxide absorption circuit is also very liable to develop a leak. This is because it contains up to 17 items which have to be joined together. If all components are not pushed home firmly, it is not uncommon for leaks to develop and, for this reason, all joints should be pressed home securely before bringing the circuit into use. Another source of leakage in a carbon dioxide circuit is failure to screw home securely the soda lime container. An unusual form of leakage can occur if a unidirectional valve becomes warped or placed off-centre so that it does not close at the appropriate moment and allows gases to pass in the wrong direction. Such abnormalities should be noticed during the routine pre-anaesthetic checking of the circuit.


## 10.6  Mechanical Ventilators

Inclusion of a mechanical ventilator in anaesthetic apparatus is a very common practice. Many varieties exist, all of which involve some kind of hazard, but the commonest hazard of all is *inexperience* on the part of the operator with the particular model. No anaesthetist, however experienced, should use an unfamiliar mechanical ventilator, for equally satisfactory anaesthesia can always be obtained by use of manual inflation. When a ventilator is in use, constant observation of the patient is vital to ensure both that the lungs are actually inflating and that oxygen and anaesthetic gases are reaching the patient. Most ventilators can *appear* to be working normally yet they may not be inflating the lungs because of disconnection of tubing between the patient and the ventilator. Although absence of inflation pressure as seen on the pressure gauge should draw attention to this, certain pressure-controlled ventilators do not possess a gauge and can continue to appear, from the noise they make, to be operating quite satisfactorily, yet no gases are reaching the patient at all.

The same defect exists in certain combined ventilator and anaesthetic apparatus, for example the Cape and the East Radcliffe. They can appear to be working normally with gases passing through the flowmeters, yet be failing to deliver oxygen and anaesthetic to the patient because the gases are passing out through the high-flow circuit and have not been diverted to the ventilator circuit. Although the machines can entrain atmospheric air in these circumstances, if an absorber is in use and the circuit closed, there will only be need to entrain sufficient air to replace the carbon dioxide extracted from the exhaled air, and this is only about 200 ml/min. As everybody knows, 200 ml air/min does not contain enough oxygen to support life. If such a machine carries a pressure gauge and if air is being entrained, a marked negative pressure phase occurs, and this should help to detect this fault—which of course should not occur if the proper checks are made before bringing the machine into use.

The Manley Pulmovent is a commonly used anaesthetic apparatus in Great Britain, driven by anaesthetic gases and oxygen. Reports of failure to inflate in spite of generous gas flow have been made: apparently inflation stopped without any warning. According to the manufacturers, who have made detailed tests, the most probable cause is a leak in the gas delivery circuit, probably the connector at the gas feed mount where the plug has not been firmly pushed home. This is another example of the benefits that could accrue from the use of clip connectors.

## 10.7  Safety Checklist

Most, if not all, of the hazards described can be avoided by instituting a routine check of apparatus before use. A draft suggestion for United States Standards includes a list of safety and performance tests which should be carried out before using any machine, and which should be affixed to the apparatus in a prominent position. The list should include the following items:

1) See that all flowmeters are closed.

2) Check pressures of 'in use' and 'full' oxygen and nitrous oxide cylinders.

3) Check correct functioning of the oxygen failure safety mechanisms.

4) If on a pipeline supply, close the reserve gas cylinders and check.

5) Open the flowmeters and check they function properly.

6) Check the level of agents in the vaporisers, adding more if necessary. When more than one vaporiser is in series, check the filler caps and see that the controls of both are closed. Empty any which the anaesthetist does not intend to use.

7) Check the emergency oxygen flushing device.

8) Check the breathing system connections—pop-off valves, unidirectional valves and coaxial circuits. Fill the system with gases and check for leaks.

9) Check the freshness or otherwise of the carbon dioxide absorbing granules in the absorber and see that the screw closing the canister is fully and tightly turned.

## 10.8  Infected Apparatus

There have been repeated demonstrations of the presence of pathogenic organisms in anaesthetic apparatus. Anaesthetic circuits, humidifiers, and ventilators have all been incriminated. There is less agreement about how far or often contamination from machines actually passes to the patient. At one time, the antibacterial properties of antistatic rubber and the filtering capacity of soda lime were thought significant, but this has been disproved. There is no doubt that organisms can pass and spread along anaesthetic tubing, but even so, to what extent such organisms cause clinical infection has not been unequivocally demonstrated. Nevertheless, ill patients have a lowered resistance; some premedicant drugs dry up secretions of the upper respiratory tract. There is need therefore to arrange for regular cleaning of all anaesthetic equipment and to insist on sterility of all equipment which passes beyond the mouth of a patient. There are several methods of sterilising anaesthetic tubing and masks:

1) *Chemical*—soaking in activated glutaraldehyde (Cidex); subsequent washing in water to remove the irritant properties of the agent is necessary.

2) *Heat sterilisation*—full autoclaving makes synthetic rubber very hard and difficult to handle. Simple immersion in nearly boiling water or low-pressure autoclaving appears more suitable. A one-step washing machine has also been described.

3) *Ethylene oxide*—exposure to ethylene oxide in a special chamber or tent is of particular value in sterilisation of ventilators which have been used on infected patients. The method is expensive and time-consuming. Nevertheless, any piece of apparatus can be treated with this method, and those hospitals that are fortunate to have such equipment can use it very widely to keep their equipment completely clean. Items such as endotracheal tubes or airways are usually passed through the central sterile supply department and returned wrapped in sterile paper.

# 11 Fires, Explosions and Electric Shock

Accurate information about the incidence of accidents from electrical equipment, or from fires and explosions in operating theatres is scanty, largely because of reluctance to publish from fear of litigation. Reports vary from an average of one death per year in the United Kingdom to 1200 in the United States. The most accurate account emanates from Australia, where an official inquiry showed that over a period of 15 years, 164 fatalities had occurred.

Operating suites contain considerable electrical equipment capable of generating sparks and causing electric shock, including fixed and portable lighting, electrically operated suction apparatus, operating tables, drills for orthopaedic work, portable X-ray equipment and image intensifiers. In addition there is equipment specifically concerned with patient treatment, which includes diathermy apparatus, heating blankets, humidifiers, blood warming equipment, electrically operated ventilators, and aids for observation of vital signs, such as cardioscopes, electrical blood pressure recorders and electrical thermometers. Recommendations for the specification, installation and maintenance of all such electrical equipment are laid down in Safety Code published by the Department of Health and Social Security. This includes instructions to all hospital authorities to appoint a senior electrical safety officer, to whom all items of electrical equipment should be referred before coming into use, to ensure that they conform to recommended specifications and are installed in a proper way. Careful observation of the Safety Code has, without doubt, reduced the incidence of accidents; nevertheless, accidents do occur from time to time.

## 11.1  Fires and Explosions

### 11.1.1  Sources

Fires and explosions in operating theatres may arise from sparks emanating from faultily installed or maintained electrical equipment, including X-ray and diathermy apparatus, as well as from sparks of static electricity, or the use of diathermy or actual cautery.

The vapours of ether and cyclopropane will catch fire at a temperature of 180°C or above. But mixture with oxygen increases the degree of flammability 200 times, so that ignition is now accompanied by a pressure change and constitutes an explosion. Being heavier than air, mixtures of cyclopropane or ether and oxygen fall to floor level, where they constitute a hazard from a lighted match or casually thrown cigarette end.

Other sources of fire include spirit burners, overheated light bulbs, disinfectant solutions containing alcohol, smoking equipment, such as cigarettes, matches and lighters, and finally patients' clothing.

Chlorhexidine in spirit is a commonly used skin disinfectant. Serious burns have followed the application of cautery to a patient's cervix after previous swabbing of the vagina with an alcoholic solution. Fire can arise from towels and swabs impregnated with alcohol and is difficult to detect, because the flame of burning alcohol is almost invisible and the first warning of its presence may be burning towels or flesh.

Several types of synthetic fibre are highly flammable and patients should always wear less inflammable cotton operating gowns in operating theatres. This recommendation is liable to be overlooked during day-patient surgery, unless particular attention is drawn to it.

A rare cause of fire, but a very lethal one, is spontaneous ignition of oil or grease in contact with compressed oxygen or air cylinder valves or pressure regulators. This occurred in an operating theatre where two operations were being carried out. The resulting explosion killed three out of four doctors and seriously injured others as well as killing the patients.

### 11.1.2  Prevention

The Safety Code deals in some detail with maintenance of electrical equipment and installation of electrical switches. Switches must never be less than 1 m above floor level. Sparks can arise from loose contacts at the light source or on equipment, as well as from worn cables. When loose contacts are suspected or cable wear is detected, the apparatus should be withdrawn from service, until the electrical safety officer has time to inspect it.

Because of their flammability, ether and cyclopropane are contra-indicated during procedures on the head and neck that involve the use of cautery, or during endoscopic procedures with battery-powered light sources. The concentration of oxygen and anaesthetic vapour persists up to 25 cm from the surface of the patient's head. Beyond this distance, however, the oxygen concentration does not exceed that of atmospheric air. Accumulation of flammable anaesthetic vapours on operating theatre floors can be prevented by installation of proper ventilating systems, with 5 to 10 changes of air per hour. In hospitals where scavenging equipment has been installed (see Chap. 9), the danger of fire and explosions from volatile anaesthetics is eliminated.

## 11.2  Static Electricity

The risk of fire or explosion from sparks produced by discharge of static electricity has been almost completely eliminated in Great Britain, by the adoption of the following measures:

1) Avoidance of hot dry atmospheres in operating suites, such as may occur if central heating is left fully on in an operating theatre with no ventilation. The probability of static charges accumulating in these conditions is very real, but can be neutralised by increasing the humidity, by spraying water on the theatre floor. Installation of proper ventilating systems with regular changes of air can eliminate this risk entirely.

2) Installation of antistatic floors in all operating suites.

3) Use of carbon-impregnated antistatic or conductive rubber on all anaesthetic apparatus. In practice conductive rubber becomes non-conductive after about 3 months. However, dampness will ensure that there is no accumulation of static charges and for this reason endo-tracheal tubes continue to be made of a red non-conductive rubber. No accidents have been reported since 1956, following the adoption of these precautions.

## 11.3  Diathermy and Cautery

Burns arising from contact between alcoholic skin disinfectants and cautery and diathermy have already been mentioned. Burns may also occur from poor contact between a diathermy electrode and the patient's skin, especially with the older heavy lead electrode, for which a wet cover or liberal use of lubricating paste is essential. The modern diathermy electrode, which is light, flexible and a better conductor, seems to have eliminated most of these problems. Another cause of burns is diathermy needles left on towels or the patient's skin whilst the foot pedal continues to make contact. Careless use of the 'actual' cautery is another cause of damage to patients' skin.

## 11.4 Electrical Equipment

Of recent years the increased use of electrical diagnostic and therapeutic devices has created a slight, but nevertheless real hazard for patients. Internal body electrodes, e.g. pacemakers, cardiac catheters and cardiac tip transducers, increase the risk of ventricular fibrillation because they have by-passed the surface of the body and its impedance or resistance qualities. Although a current of 80-100 mA is necessary to induce ventricular fibrillation through the skin, a much smaller current of 80 $\mu$A is hazardous to a normal human heart from electrical equipment inside the body. Transducers are said to offer an unrivalled opportunity for ventricular fibrillation should faults develop. Attention to careful construction and regular expert maintenance and testing before each use are the best ways of avoiding accidents from these sources.

### 11.4.1 Endoscopes
Endoscopes are often connected to low-voltage battery equipment. It is dangerous to use more than one endoscope from one power source. A fatality has been reported from the simultaneous use of two endoscopes connected to the same source of low voltage; the patient was electrocuted.

### 11.4.2 Thermometers
Electrical thermometers are of two types—thermistors (temperature transducers) and thermocouples. Although battery-operated instruments (low voltage) are safer, most are mains-operated and must be carefully earthed and the metal probes plastic-coated to prevent inadvertent burns to oesophagus or rectum during the use of diathermy.

### 11.4.3 Pacemakers
Patients with heart block will require anaesthesia (a) for insertion of the pacemakers, (b) for surgery for other conditions, (c) for temporary pacing during and after surgery. When undertaking these procedures, an intravenous drip is absolutely essential, together with a solution of isoprenaline (2-4 mg/litre in 5% dextrose) which can be diverted into the drip to maintain cardiac contractions during insertion or change of the pacemakers.

The use of surgical diathermy and other radio-frequency apparatus such as a powerful walkie-talkie, is dangerous in the neighbourhood of such patients and carries risk of ventricular fibrillation. The guidelines for their use should be carefully followed.

### 11.4.4 Blood Warmers
Usually blood is warmed by passage through a plastic coil immersed in a water bath whose temperature is kept constant at 37°C by a thermostatically controlled electric element. The main hazards are overheating

and faulty earthing. Overheating from failure of the thermostat can be detected by the inclusion of an accurate thermometer in the water bath in an easily seen position. To prevent shorting, the metal stand on the warmer should be bonded to the EPR system.

### 11.4.5 ECG Equipment

Monitoring of the electrocardiograph is used with increasing frequency in routine anaesthesia. In many American units the cardioscope is a standard piece of equipment. The electrical equipment inside the cardioscope is very carefully insulated by the casing and the input from the patient is also carefully separated from the amplifying equipment. Hence, ECG apparatus carries very little hazard, compared with smaller and less sophisticated pieces of equipment, such as electrical suction apparatus and blood warmers, which do not receive the same supervision and servicing as cardioscopes. Loose plugs and worn insulating material on the cables, exposing the wires underneath, are more commonly causes of electric shocks.

# 12 Induction

## 12.1  Preliminaries

Before discussing the pitfalls of actual induction of anaesthesia, certain preliminary procedures deserve attention. A routine must be established to prevent anaesthetising the wrong patient or performing of the wrong operation. Although anaesthetists are not solely responsible they are part of a series of checking procedures, which includes nurses and surgeons, designed to ensure that errors do not occur.

In most hospitals an identification routine precedes induction of anaesthesia:

1) The identity of the patient can be established from the identity band, which should of course coincide with the clinical notes.

2) The patient's name and the nature of the operation in the clinical record should coincide with the operation list in the operating theatre; if a left- or right-sided procedure is to be undertaken, it is a wise precaution to ask the patient, 'Which side?'

3) The patient's record should show time of administration of premedication and the signature of the nurse responsible. Failure to administer premedication can increase the hazards of subsequent anaesthesia.

4) It is a nursing duty to remove dentures before patients come to the operating suite, but anaesthetists should check this as well as taking note of bridgework or crowned teeth.

5) A signed form of consent to operation is essential to protect surgeon and anaesthetist, for if proper consent has not been given, induction of anaesthesia and surgery may constitute grounds for a charge of 'assault'. Minors (under 18 years of age) may sign their own consent form if of sufficient intelligence to understand what is to occur.

In emergency situations, in addition to the above, enquiry must be made about the time and nature of the last meal. The procedure to follow in the event of a positive answer is set out in Chap. 25.

Although the above procedures take a few minutes, their routine observation on *every* patient would reduce litigation arising from mistakes in identity and from performance of the wrong operation, or operating on the wrong side.

## 12.2 Intravenous Induction

### 12.2.1 Preparation of Solutions

Some intravenous agents are manufactured already dissolved and only need transfer from ampoule to syringe. Others however, notably the barbiturates, require dissolving a measured quantity in sterile water. Anaesthetists are responsible for the effects of any substance injected and should never use solutions prepared by some other person unless satisfied that they contain the anaesthetic required in correct strength. Deaths have occurred from intravenous injection of cetrimide and halothane, drawn up from multidose bottles supposed to contain thiopentone solution.

### 12.2.2 Selection of Suitable Veins

In many patients, selection of a suitable vein presents difficulties. There are three common sites—the antecubital fossa, the forearm, and the back of the hand. Each has its advantages and disadvantages.

The *antecubital fossa* offers two prominent veins, the median cephalic and median basilic. In most patients the bicipital fascia covers most of the ulnar artery in the antecubital fossa, but in over 10% of patients it runs downwards and inwards in a sloping manner, leaving around 3 cm of the ulnar artery visible and in direct contact with the median basilic vein, whose use for induction carries a high risk of intra-arterial injection. On rare occasions the ulnar artery takes an abnormal course, passing in front of the bicipital fascia over the forearm in a leash of branches very similar in appearance to veins, for which they can easily be mistaken, offering a second site for an intra-arterial injection. Puncturing of veins on the inner side of the arm or the antecubital fossa should be preceded by palpation to ensure that an artery is not present.

The median nerve in the antecubital fossa lies just under the median basilic and cephalic veins and the brachial artery where it divides into radial and ulnar branches, thus within reach of anaesthetic agents injected outside a vein.

*Forearm veins* are not prominent and lie a little deeper than those on the dorsum of the hand. They are surprisingly easy to puncture because they are well anchored to the fascia and do not slide to one side in the presence of an advancing needle.

The radial vein at the lower end just above the wrist, although usually reserved for intravenous infusions, can also be used for simple intravenous injections. Owing to the radial nerve's presence deep to the vein, extravenous injection of irritant solutions or too deep a passage of the needle can cause damage.

The lateral and median cutaneous nerves run down on either side of the forearm and are susceptible to extravenous injection of irritant solutions. They can be best avoided by confining punctures to veins in the mid-position.

The veins on the *back of the hand* are prominent and offer an invitation to insert a small butterfly scalp vein needle, thus securing permanent access to a vein throughout the operation. Formation of haematomas and discoloration of the skin from bruising are disadvantages and cause more after-pain than vein puncture elsewhere in the arm.

The posterior branch of the radial artery runs through the 'anatomical snuff box' between the first and second metatarsals on the back of the hand. When the main artery takes this course, its prominence may lead to confusion with a vein. This can be avoided by palpation before attempting puncture of this part of the hand.

### 12.2.3 Difficulties in Vein Puncture

Whilst repeated failure to enter a vein is not, strictly speaking, a 'hazard', it can distress a patient and embarrass an operator. Patients with poor peripheral circulation never have prominent veins, and in others (especially those with surplus subcutaneous fat) veins are deeply placed and difficult to see. Frightened or shocked patients also have constricted veins.

There are several ways of improving dilation of constricted or poorly visible veins. One of the less well advertised benefits of good pre-operative sedation is a warm, relaxed patient with dilated veins. Veins are often more prominent on the arm which is most commonly used, so enquiry as to whether a patient is right- or left-handed can be helpful. Light friction and rubbing helps dilation of the veins. This is not an 'old wives' tale' but an established physiological fact. If these measures fail, application of warmth, preferably by an electrical heating pad for a few minutes, may improve the filling of the veins. Sometimes small super-ficial veins are visible on the anterior aspect of the wrist. Attempts to enter them should only be made with a small sharp needle, for the area is particularly sensitive.

It is inadvisable to attempt more than three punctures with the same needle, since the point becomes blunted.

If an intravenous infusion is a necessary preliminary to surgery, as for example in shocked patients, vasodilation follows intramuscular injection of 25 mg chlorpromazine in about 15 min. Alternatively, inhalation of halothane (see Sect. 12.5.6) improves peripheral circulation, with appearance of prominent veins.

No anaesthetist should be afraid to admit failure. If three or four efforts on each arm are unsuccessful, patients usually welcome an inhalation induction.

## 12.3  Intravenous Anaesthetic Agents

Intravenous induction agents are the barbiturate derivatives thiopentone, methohexitone and hexobarbitone and the non-barbiturates alphaxalone and alphadolone, ketamine and etomidate.

### 12.3.1  Thiopentone

Thiopentone (Pentothal, Intraval) has been in constant use since 1935. For at least ten years after its introduction it was often used as the sole anaesthetic for major surgery. In 1942 nearly 7000 major operations were performed under thiopentone, alone or with local analgesia, in the Mayo Clinic. The average dose was 1.5-2.0 g (two to three times what is current practice) and 3 g was by no means uncommon. Compared with these figures, doses in current use appear almost homoeopathic. Of course the administration of these large amounts was by intermittent doses of 100-200 mg over a period of hours rather than minutes. Surprisingly the hazards and complications of smaller doses differ little from those encountered following a large intermittent dosage, except that prolonged recovery and postoperative respiratory depression no longer occur. Hazards arising from present-day use of thiopentone as an induction agent can be divided into local and general.

*Local Hazards.* Apart from complications common to any intravenous injection (infection, haematoma formation, damage to nerve, loss of a broken needle), thiopentone carries additional hazards arising from subcutaneous and arterial injection.

Subcutaneous injection of 5% solutions can be followed by cellulitis and slough formation, but since the adoption of 2.5% solutions, tissue damage after subcutaneous injection does not occur.

Intra-arterial injection of 5% solution remains a major hazard, although the 2.5% solution is said not to cause adverse complications. Intra-arterial injection is accompanied by immediate complaint of severe pain comparable to that following plunging the arm into boiling water. Visible signs are blanching and cyanosis of the hand from temporary arterial spasm and the release of noradrenaline. Contrary to common belief, arterial spasm is not the main cause of ischaemia and gangrene of the fingers following arterial injection. The real cause is thrombosis from the crystallisation of thiopentone at the normal pH of plasma in the blood vessels. Damage to the endothelial and subendothelial tissue causes formation of thrombi. These changes are not a consequence of the pH of the thiopentone solution, because they do not occur following intra-arterial injection of an alkaline solution of pH 10.6, the same as thiopentone.

The needle should be left in the artery for injection of a vasodilator such as tolazoline (Priscol) 30 mg, an antispasmodic such as papaverine 40-30 mg in 20 ml saline, and heparin 3 mg/kg to prevent thrombus formation. Heparin may also be given intravenously. Brachial plexus block is also recommended.

*General Hazards.* These are related to the circulation and the respiratory system, to hypersensitivity, and to shock, haemorrhage and dehydration.

*Circulatory Hazards.* A dose of 500 mg or less of thiopentone is unlikely to have any serious direct depressant action on heart muscle of the average patient. Following induction, circulatory response is minimal if the dosage is confined to the sleep dose (the amount required to abolish consciousness) plus half that amount, which ensures 5-10 min of unconsciousness, ample for the subsequent inhalation maintenance agent to become effective.

Fall in systolic blood pressure in hypertensive subjects is greater than in normotensives, since thiopentone tends to convert a hypertensive to a normotensive state, but compensatory increase of cardiac output ensures peripheral and coronary perfusion. The presence of known circulatory impairment is a contra-indication to the administration of thiopentone, because weakness of cardiac muscle or presence of aortic stenosis or constrictive pericarditis prevents increase of cardiac output after decrease of peripheral resistance, and coronary circulation becomes inadequate.

*Respiratory Complications.* Thiopentone is an acknowledged respiratory depressant, and hence its use is contra-indicated in the presence of respiratory obstruction due either to inflammatory and neoplastic conditions or to depression of muscular activity occurring in muscle dystrophies, and in the presence of porphyria or nervous demyelinisation. In the average subject, the extent of depression following intravenous administration is directly related to the amount of opiate in the preoperative medication. Loss of consciousness is accompanied by hyperventilation, which eliminates carbon dioxide and explains the ensuing brief apnoea. If no more than half the sleep dose is added, respiration resumes within a few seconds, but it remains rather shallow after opiate premedication. The administration of more thiopentone than this carries a risk of more profound depression of respiration—which will, however, respond to a strong surgical stimulus.

Hiccup, obstructed airway and laryngospasm are frequent respiratory complications following thiopentone and can with some justification be defined as adverse reactions since they have existed since the first days of thiopentone and no sure means of their avoidance has been devised in 35 years.

Hiccupping may occur following induction and may persist intermittently for several minutes. Though not a cause for concern, it has considerable nuisance value. Its duration can be shortened by inhalation of carbon dioxide, which also deepens respiration.

Obstruction of the airway by the tongue falling back into the pharynx can complicate any anaesthetic but it has particular significance following thiopentone. Pulling the jaw forward (and with it the tongue) *should* clear the airway for resumption of respiration after the period of apnoea. Sometimes this manoeuvre is not successful and although respiratory efforts appear to resume, seen as retraction of the lower ribs, no air enters the chest. Inexperienced anaesthetists, because they concentrate on chest movements rather than those of the reservoir bag, do not always appreciate the presence of obstruction until cyanosis causes marked circulatory depression, sufficient on occasion to lead to cardiac arrest. Patients with dark skins are at additional risk because in them cyanosis is not so easily detected. To avoid such errors during the period of apnoea, gentle pressure should be applied to the inflated reservoir bag. If air does not enter the lungs freely, the jaw should be pulled forward once more and a pharyngeal airway inserted, although this may cause laryngospasm.

Laryngospasm is the most consistent and troublesome complication of thiopentone. It is impossible to predict the occurrence of this complication but it should be anticipated in plethoric subjects, heavy drinkers and smokers, and sufferers from chronic bronchitis. Its onset often coincides with the few deep breaths that accompany the onset of anaesthesia. On other occasions, cough and spasm occur after induction for no obvious cause (possibly from a fleck of mucus on the vocal cords), or after premature insertion of an airway.

Laryngospasm is an alarming experience and calls for a cool head and careful application of simple principles to obtain a clear airway. After pulling the jaw forward, one holds the face mask firmly in place and maintains gentle pressure on the reservoir bag (inflated with oxygen), so that even after a small respiratory effort, some oxygen passes through the partially closed vocal cords, whilst progressive rise in the carbon dioxide level of the bloodstream has an antispasmodic effect and stimulates breathing. Heavy opiate premedication reduces the sensitivity of the respiratory centre to carbon dioxide and will delay resumption of breathing. A time limit should be set for this condition to correct itself, and if no improvement occurs after, say, 60 s, a quick-acting relaxant (suxamethonium or fazadinium) should be injected. Immediate relief of spasm allows passage of an endotracheal tube and control of bronchial irritability by inflation with an inhalational anaesthetic.

Some anaesthetists believe that laryngospasm occurs more commonly when too small a dose of thiopentone has been given. The incidence is said to be reduced when a small dose (40 mg) of gallamine is added to 0.5 g thiopentone. The inclusion of promethazine (Phenergan) in premedication also reduces the incidence.

*Hypersensitivity.* Use of thiopentone is rarely complicated by hypersensitivity and anaphylactic response, only eight cases having been reported in the literature, although many anaesthetists believe the incidence to be higher. All the cases reported had received many inductions with thiopentone, mainly for check cystoscopy after treatment of bladder tumours. The onset is sudden even after a dose as small as 100 mg. There is violent coughing and spasm of the bronchi, accompanied by cyanosis, tachycardia and circulatory collapse. Skin manifestations such as erythema and urticaria do occur. The condition must be carefully distinguished from laryngospasm. It must also be distinguished from the violent coughing of bronchitics after thiopentone or following surgical stimulus. Intravenous promethazine 25 mg often relieves this coughing, and can also be given as prophylaxis when past experience suggests the need for it.

## 12.3.2 Methohexitone

When first synthesised, methohexitone (Brietal) was discarded as an intravenous anaesthetic because of its brief action. However, demand for an agent with rapid action, minimal cardiac and respiratory depression and rapid recovery led to its reintroduction and it has earned considerable popularity. The main hazard, when it is used as an induction agent, is early recovery of consciousness in resistant subjects, before the absorption of sufficient of the inhalational maintenance agent. The incidence of hiccup, sneezing and coughing is also higher than after thiopentone.

## 12.3.3 Hexobarbitone

Hexobarbitone (Evipan) closely resembles thiopentone, except that involuntary muscle movement and hiccup are more frequent and the duration of anaesthesia is shorter.

### 12.3.4   Alphaxalone and Alphadolone

The combination of these agents (Althesin) is a steroid anaesthetic to which polyoxyethylated castor oil has been added to increase its solubility in water. Rapid undepressed recovery suggests it could have a very useful place in out-patient and day surgery. Progress has been curtailed by the incidence of undesirable side-effects—1:2000—most of which are anaphylactoid in nature, and some of which have been fatal. Strong doubts have been expressed about its suitability for general use, unless the use of other agents is positively contra-indicated.

### 12.3.5   Ketamine

Though not strictly an induction agent, ketamine (Ketalar) can be used for this purpose, especially in paediatric anaesthesia when difficulties present themselves in the form of emotional parents.

Ketamine administered by intravenous or intramuscular injection induces a state of anaesthesia which preserves the protective laryngeal reflexes and does not induce cardiovascular depression. However, unwelcome side-effects have been reported. During anaesthesia, failure to tolerate surgical stimuli, increased bleeding and increase in muscle tone have been observed, and in more than a third of the patients, vocalisation and purposeful movements of the limbs and head occurred.

Recovery is often accompanied by disorganisation of the central nervous system, in children as well as in adults, with disorientation and hallucinations causing serious emotional disturbance. In children restlessness, disorientation and crying have all been observed, as has prolongation of the recovery period after intramuscular injection. Preservation of laryngeal reflexes has also been questioned. Radio-opaque material placed in the pharynx has been shown to enter the trachea after intravenous dose of 4-5 mg ketamine/kg, although in children similar doses have been reported to increase laryngeal sensitivity and cause laryngospasm. This is not so surprising, because the laryngeal reflexes in the very young are much more sensitive and much more difficult to depress than in adults.

Side-effects during recovery can be prevented by separation from other patients in a quiet area, so that outside stimuli are kept to a minimum. Drugs with a deafferenting action given as premedication or at the end of the operation also help significantly to reduce emergence phenomena. Chlorpromazine or diazepam given intramuscularly in appropriate dosage has been recommended.

### 12.3.6   Diazepam

Strictly speaking, diazepam (Valium) is a hypnotic with pronounced amnesic properties and little analgesic action. No depression of respiration or the cardiovascular system occurs following its administration. It is considered a suitable induction agent for poor-risk elderly subjects.

Hazards include pain during injection, especially in small veins, followed by thrombosis as a late complication (48-72 h) and thus not seen by anaesthetists. Difficulties may be experienced in maintenance with inhalational agents after induction (coughing, spasm and salivation, particularly after trichloroethylene and ether), especially if sufficient time is not allowed for the diazepam to become effective (at least 5-10 min). Diazepam reduces muscle tone and increases threefold the neuro-muscular relaxant properties of non-depolarising relaxants—hence they must be used with great caution. Diazepam crosses the placental barrier and is therefore not recommended in obstetric practice. The metabolism of diazepam is uncertain, but as both the liver and kidneys appear to be involved, failure of these organs constitutes a contra-indication to its use.

### 13.3.7 Etomidate

Etomidate is a recently introduced non-barbiturate intravenous anaes-thetic derived from imidazole carboxylate whose advertised advantages are cardiovascular stability and lack of irritant or histamine-releasing properties. The recommended dose is 0.3 mg/kg or 20 g for a 70-kg adult. So far, it has been used in trials on out-patients. The hazards or drawbacks differ very little from other intravenous agents. There is a fairly high incidence of involuntary muscle movement during uncon-sciousness, but as in the case of the early barbiturates, this can be reduced to tolerable levels by opiate premedication. Pain sometimes occurs on injection, and more often when small veins are used. The speed of injection also seems to be significant: the faster it is injected, the less the pain. Respiratory disturbances similar to those seen in other short-acting intravenous agents include hiccup, coughing and laryngospasm, with a frequency neither much more nor much less than other agents. On recovery, nausea and vomiting occur with greater frequency than after thiopentone, and would seem to bear no relation to the dose admin-istered. This agent is not regarded as particularly suitable for short out-patient procedures, because satisfactory anaesthesia free from involun-tary muscle movement cannot be obtained without heavy opiate premedication.

## 12.4 Inhalational Induction

Induction by an inhalational method is probably the safest for the patient because the anaesthetist retains control: the anaesthetic gases enter and leave the patient's circulation by a physical process independent of metabolic activity. Nevertheless, it is seldom undertaken in adults unless intravenous induction is contra-indicated. There are, of course, exceptions. Elderly and feeble subjects, for whom rapid recovery and mobilisation following inhalational anaesthesia are distinct advantages seldom object to inhalational induction. Otherwise, inhalational induction is confined to young children, especially those for whom the needle holds more terror than an anaesthetic face mask. Adults still receive inhalational induction in dental surgery but it has largely been replaced by local analgesia or intravenous anaesthesia using metho-hexitone with an inhalational supplement.

### 12.4.1 Secretions

All inhalational agents increase the flow of saliva, hence premedication must always include a drying agent such as atropine or hyoscine. In recent years, phenothiazines and other antihistamines have been shown to provide satisfactory drying properties in addition to their tranquillizing and anti-emetic actions.

### 12.4.2 Excitement Phase

Induction of anaesthesia with intravenous agents is so rapid that the struggling phase at the transition to unconsciousness is no longer visible. With inhalational agents, which are slower in action, excitement does occur; it is scarcely noticeable with rapid-acting cyclopropane, but very evident with slower-acting ether.

The duration of the struggling phase can be reduced by a speedy induction. Depression of respiration after opiate premedication reduces the speed of induction. Omission of opiates and inclusion of a little carbon dioxide in the inhaled mixture hasten induction with all inhalational agents and shorten the excitement phase.

### 12.4.3 Vomiting

Vomiting can occur during inhalational induction, particularly with ether. It is often the result of severe coughing due to the irritant nature of the vapour. As it occurs before the patient is unconscious, protective reflexes remain intact. Usually it is preceded by breath-holding and a swallowing movement. If these occur, the patient should be turned immediately into the lateral position with the head lowered, so that if vomiting occurs the vomit will flow out of the mouth. During the act of vomiting, respiration is inhibited, so that keeping the head low avoids any danger of inhalation. If the mask is held on the face and the patient remains supine, vomiting will be followed by inhalation into the trachea. The patient should remain in the lateral position as the induction continues.

## 12.5  Inhalational Induction Agents

### 12.5.1 Nitrous Oxide

The chief disadvantage of nitrous oxide is lack of potency, which in the past has led to the exclusion of oxygen from the inspired mixture to a dangerous extent. The resulting cerebral anoxia from time to time caused permanent brain damage. Nitrous oxide is now never used in such a manner; at least 20% oxygen is always added.

The weak anaesthetic properties of nitrous oxide can be supplemented by intravenous opiates. Pethidine was popular in the past and is now largely replaced by neuroleptanalgesic techniques (Sect. 16.5.2). Inhalational agents in low concentrations are also effective.

### 12.5.2  Cyclopropane

The highly inflammable and explosive properties of cyclopropane and the availability of non-inflammable anaesthetic agents have led to a significant reduction in use of this agent. Rapid induction and the large percentage of oxygen in the inhaled mixture are reasons for its use in emergency and poor-risk surgery. Because of its inflammability and its cost, it is always used with carbon dioxide absorption techniques. As vagal tone is increased by cyclopropane, premedication with atropine is necessary to prevent bradycardia. Ventricular extrasystoles are commonly encountered, possibly due to carbon dioxide accumulation but more likely to sympathetic activity, since deepening of the anaesthesia reduces incidence. The peripheral vessels are dilated and bleeding is increased with cyclopropane anaesthesia. Since cyclopropane, like ether, is a sympathetic stimulant, blood pressure is well maintained during its administration.

Cyclopropane raises the blood sugar and is contra-indicated in the presence of diabetes mellitus.

Diathermy or cautery must never be used when the patient is receiving cyclopropane (see Sect. 11.1).

### 12.5.3  Ether

Inflammability in air and explosiveness in oxygen are the major hazards of ether vapour, rendering it unsuitable for use with diathermy or cautery, or during endoscopy procedures in mouth, trachea or bronchi when the light source is an illuminating bulb (the hazard does not arise when a fibre-optic light source is in use). The vapour is irritant, causing coughing and spasm and mucous secretion, particularly unpleasant for sufferers from chronic bronchitis. Induction with ether is said to be long and tedious, but this is true only if respiration is depressed after opiate premedication. Reasonably rapid induction with ether follows pre-medication which avoids opiates, if the induction technique includes partial rebreathing or the inclusion of a little carbon dioxide in the inspired mixture.

Clinically, ether does not depress the heart or respiration. An apparent cardiac stimulant effect results from sympathetic stimulation, although ether itself has a direct depressant effect upon the heart. Whilst there is no direct depressant effect on the respiratory centre following an overdose, respiration stops before the heart beat, as with other inhalational anaesthetics. During recovery, nausea and vomiting occur commonly. Irritation of the air passages is said to cause an increased incidence of postoperative pulmonary atelectasis.

In bygone days it was common practice to give ether with nitrous oxide and oxygen, using some apparatus of the Boyle's type, because it was thought that with this method the patient received as little ether as possible. No-one has ever proved this, and in fact the nitrous oxide/oxygen/ether induction is one of the most difficult to undertake with success, and has been responsible for many accidents in the past. If it is decided to use ether for reasons of economy or convenience, the best method is to use an Oxford vaporiser. With this machine, the quantity of ether the patient receives can be controlled and excellent operating conditions provided.

### 12.5.4 Trichloroethylene

Trichloroethylene is mainly used in anaesthesia for its analgesic properties, which are effective at low concentrations of the drug. It is often used as a supplementary agent during nitrous oxide and oxygen anaesthesia. Rapid breathing or tachypnoea may occur during anaesthesia with trichloroethylene; this can be reduced by intravenous administration of small amounts of an opiate (e.g. pethidine).

Bradycardia or slow pulse sometimes occur if premedication with atropine is omitted. Extrasystoles may occur, and adrenaline should never be used in conjunction with trichloroethylene, as the myocardium is said to be sensitised to its effects, thus carrying the risk of ventricular fibrillation (see, however, comments on halothane below, Sect. 12.5.6).

Trichloroethylene should never be used in a closed circuit, since when the vapour passes through soda lime, a toxic substance, dichloroacetylene, may be formed.

### 12.5.5 Methoxyflurane

Methoxyflurane, a halogenated compound, is a recent addition to anaesthetic agents. Because of its low volatility, induction is slow, taking about 8 min to achieve full narcosis. No very serious cardiovascular effects have been reported, although in deep anaesthesia the myocardium is said to be depressed.

Breakdown products of methoxyflurane (inorganic fluoride) can accumulate in the kidney, causing obstruction of the tubules. The concentration of fluoride does not reach a critical level unless administration exceeds 2 h. The level of toxicity is said to be increased when tetracyclines are administered at the same time as the anaesthetic.

Transaminase studies in man have not provided any evidence of toxic effects on the liver. Four fatal cases of liver necrosis have been reported following the use of methoxyflurane, but it would be unwise in the lack of any other evidence to attribute this to the anaesthetic itself. Methoxy-flurane causes a rise in blood sugar and therefore should not be used in patients with severe diabetes.

### 12.5.6  Halothane

It could be said with some truth that halothane is the victim of its own excellence. The introduction of halothane into clinical anaesthesia took place in England in 1956, after 26 years' research, and was preceded by a detailed study of its effect on many species of animal. Within a few years it was estimated that over 75% of patients anaesthetised in Great Britain received halothane. The rapid spread of the use of this agent must have had a serious effect on the sale of other agents, whose manufacturers did not fail to draw attention to any faults or hazards of halothane which arose in the literature, to the advantage of their own products. Thus a considerable number of halothane hazards have been described; most are avoidable by careful administration and others (e.g. hepatotoxicity) are not thought by everyone to be real.

Halothane has been subject to criticism on several grounds: respiratory depression, poor analgesic properties, cardiac depression and increased sensitivity to adrenaline, hypotension, excessive relaxation of uterine muscle, muscular rigidity and shivering on recovery and, already mentioned, alleged hepatotoxicity.

*Respiratory Depression.* Halothane is a respiratory depressant, but under its action respiration ceases well before any serious cardio-vascular depression, whilst a surgical stimulus will always result in deeper and faster breathing. This property has been described as an 'in-built' servo or self-regulatory mechanism. To a large extent patients can control the amount of vapour they inhale through the strength of the operative stimulus, breathing deeply when pain impulses get through and automatically deepening anaesthesia. This action is well illustrated in the 'closed' halothane-oxygen technique.

When anaesthetising neonates and infants, respiratory depression can cause problems. In these small subjects breathing rapidly becomes shallow soon after induction, giving the impression of sudden deepening of the anaesthesia. The anaesthetist withdraws the agent, only to discover that the pain of the surgeon's incision evokes violent movement of the limbs, and it takes some minutes of further halothane adminis-tration before the operation can resume.

*Cardiac Effects.* Halothane is described as a direct depressant of cardiac muscle, but this property is certainly not apparent in clinical anaesthesia. It could be related to a reduction of secretion and intensity of action of noradrenaline, which is released in the sympathetic nerve terminals in heart muscle. This effect, together with a lowering of peripheral resistance from vasodilatation, without doubt reduces oxygen require-ment and could explain the reduction of damage to heart muscle observed following experimental coronary occlusion in dogs under halothane anaesthesia, compared with control animals undergoing the same procedure without halothane.

Cardiac arrhythmias occur during halothane anaesthesia and are said to arise from accumulation of carbon dioxide, the result of shallow breathing. Extrasystoles can occur for this reason during any inhalational anaesthetic and are not an exclusive feature of halothane.

*Hypotension.* Halothane reduces systolic blood pressure in several ways. Bradycardia reduces cardiac output, but is easily reversed by 0.6 g atropine. More significant is the effect of relaxation of smooth muscle in the venous and arterial systems. Besides increasing the overall capacitance of the vascular system by 25%, it also reduces peripheral resistance, both factors contributing to a fall in blood pressure. A fall in pressure nearly always occurs after induction with halothane in the absence of a surgical stimulus. Pressures around 12 kPa are not uncommon, just as they are following the reduction of sympathetic tone after spinal or epidural blocks. These pressures are acceptable since perfusion of the tissues remains adequate (see Sect. 18.1.3). Under halothane, however, a surgical stimulus quickly restores pressure to near the pre-operative level through reflex sympathetic responses.

*Action on Uterine Muscle.* Halothane, like chloroform, relaxes uterine muscle, especially as anaesthesia deepens. Before calibrated temperature-compensated vaporisers became available, Boyle's bottles were used to administer halothane and far too high a concentration was obtained. Used in this way in obstetric practice, there was a significant increase in post partum bleeding after abortion and after childbirth. This explains why many obstetricians do not like this agent for their patients. However, the introduction of calibrated vaporisers has changed the picture. It has been shown in a large series that blood loss after delivery following halothane was no greater and no less than that following the use of ether, cyclopropane or trichloroethylene. It has also been shown that uterine contractions occur twice as quickly after halothane than after ether. Although halothane passes the placental barrier, it is suitable in low concentrations for vaginal delivery and useful in higher concentrations to produce relaxation for external version or manual removal of the placenta, or to produce relaxation of a contraction ring.

*Muscle Spasticity During Recovery.* Shivering and muscle spasticity sometimes occur during recovery from halothane. This was originally thought to be a compensatory effect to a fall in body temperature from vasodilatation during surgery. A more likely explanation is that it arises from a centrally induced increase of muscle tone.

During recovery from halothane, because of the agent's poor analgesic properties, pain impulses reach the sensory cortex before full recovery in sufficient strength to set up activity in the Betz cells of the motor cortex; these send discharges down the pyramidal tract that are sufficiently intense to induce movements of the limbs. Some of these impulses doubtless enter the reticular formation through the collaterals from the pyramidal tract, where they activate the muscle facilitatory centre in the pontomedullary reticular formation, leading to an overall increase of muscle tone through the reticulospinal tracts. The effectiveness in restoring normal tone displayed by phenothiazines which deafferent the reticular formation is some measure of support for this hypothesis.

*Alleged Hepatotoxicity.* If one of halothane's misfortunes is its excellence, then its chemical similarity to chloroform (a recognised liver poison) is another. Soon after halothane became widely used in the United States, reports of postoperative jaundice, resembling viral hepatitis, in patients who had received halothane gave rise to misgivings, especially in view of this agent's chemical resemblance to chloroform.

The American National Academy of Science set up a national halothane study, which reported in 1969 their findings from a nationwide survey of many thousands of anaesthetic procedures performed with all agents available at that time. They reported that the incidence of postoperative jaundice bore no particular relation to the anaesthetic agents used, whilst mortality after surgery was lower with halothane than with any other agent. A private study on similar lines at the Mayo Clinic supported these findings.

An epidemiological study in Great Britain showed that the number of patients likely to contract viral hepatitis *by chance* after a surgical operation in the United Kingdom, or in the United States where the incidence of this infection is five times greater, was considerably less than the reported incidence of jaundice after halothane in either country. It is therefore possible that all patients developing unexplained jaundice after halothane could by chance have been incubating viral hepatitis. The irregular incubation period, varying from hours to weeks, and the identity of the pathological changes seen with those of viral hepatitis give support to this explanation.

Animal experimentation has repeatedly failed to reveal hepatotoxic properties in halothane similar to those of chloroform, alcohol or phosphorus, which consistently cause liver damage in small animals. Indeed, it has been shown that when very small amounts of these substances (one hundredth the effective intravenous dose) are placed in contact with the autonomic nerves in the portal fissure of small animals, liver necrosis is a constant finding, suggesting a possible neural background for hepatitis. The liver, like kidney and lungs, is known to be subject to vascular and other changes in response to injury, bacterial infection and chemical irritants. Changes in serum bilirubin have been shown to take place after surgery, greater in the upper abdomen than the lower, and cellular immunity to infection has also been shown to be depressed for 2-3 weeks after surgical operations.

A recent report suggested that there was an increased risk of jaundice after more than one halothane administration within a few weeks, but this has not been confirmed by later studies. Furthermore, there are many units treating burns and leukaemic conditions where patients receive halothane weekly, or at even shorter intervals, for several months with no apparent ill effects. This does not support a recent suggestion that jaundice after repeated halothane is due to the acquirement of an unrecognised type of sensitivity and is therefore a valid reason for denying halothane to any patient who has received it within the past month.

The following answer to a suggestion that fear of jaundice justifies restriction of the use of halothane in major surgery summarises the attitude of many practising anaesthetists: 'To avoid it [i.e. halothane in major surgery] implies that there are safer alternatives. This is not the case. Indeed, what studies there are of anaesthetic morbidity and mortality, suggest that halothane is probably the "safest agent" currently available.'

Nevertheless, allegations continue to be made about the hepatotoxicity of halothane and the term 'halothane hepatitis' continues to be used incorrectly as though it were a specific acknowledged pathological state, whereas to the contrary it cannot be distinguished from viral hepatitis.

To sum up, the alleged hepatotoxicity of halothane is not established and no justification exists for the use of the term 'halothane hepatitis' in any scientific department.

*Adverse Effects of Adrenaline.* There is evidence that halothane sensitizes the beta-adrenergic receptors of the heart to exogenous adrenaline, thus making the heart more liable to ventricular fibrillation following injection of adrenaline. This evidence is in conflict with the reported property of antagonising the action of noradrenaline released at the sympathetic nerve terminals in the heart muscle. There has, however, been one report of cardiac arrest in asystole, following infiltration of adrenaline during anaesthesia. In spite of this, there is widespread tolerance by anaesthetists of subcutaneous injection of adrenaline and saline diluted to strengths between 1:100 000 and 1:200 000 by surgeons in an effort to reduce bleeding during thyroidectomy and operations for pelvic prolapse. Some anaesthetists recommend the injection of a beta-blocker such as practolol 5 mg before allowing surgeons to infiltrate with adrenaline and saline. Certainly strengths greater than 1:100 000 should not be tolerated, and pressure should be put on surgeons to discontinue a practice of no great benefit and potentially hazardous to patients.

### 12.5.7 Enflurane

Enflurane (Ethrane) is yet another halogenated anaesthetic, being a fluorinated ether whose physical characteristics resemble halothane.

Although enflurane has no analgesic action before unconsciousness, muscular relaxation (as found in most ethers) sufficient for abdominal surgery is obtainable, with adequate spontaneous respiration and a normal $P_{CO_2}$.

The action of tubocurarine is intensified in a manner which is not susceptible to reversal by neostigmine, although presumably stopping administration and reducing the blood concentration would have the same effect. There is no similar action with depolarising agents such as suxamethonium.

Minimal cardiovascular changes, taken with the above-mentioned properties, suggest a useful agent. Unfortunately it may be epileptogenic. EEG tracings under enflurane may show marked wave and spike activity and epileptiform seizures have been recorded. On the other hand such changes may be delayed for up to 16 days, giving rise to a suggestion that a metabolite produces them.

Only 2.4% of this compound is excreted in the urine as fluorinated metabolites, of which only 0.5% appears as fluoride, so it should not cause renal damage. One report of hepatocellular dysfunction without jaundice has appeared.

In spite of its attractive properties, enflurane's cost and high epileptogenic activity suggest that widespread adoption of this agent is unlikely.

# 13 Muscle Relaxants

The original purpose of muscle relaxants in anaesthesia was to relax abdominal muscles during surgery without the need to saturate patients with ether. With the passage of time, the indications have expanded to include the provision of relaxation for various examinations under anaesthetic, to facilitate passage of endotracheal tubes, to allow the conduct of artificial respiration, and—by suppressing reflex movements to painful stimuli when small doses are given—to reduce the total quantity of anaesthetic needed for any particular operation.

Two main types of muscle relaxant are available: (a) competitive blockers, i.e. those that compete with acetylcholine at the neuromuscular junction; and (b) depolarising blockers, i.e. those which by mimicking the action of acetylcholine on the muscle fibre induce a permanent depolarisation and paralysis after endogenous acetylcholine (which produces depolarisation) has been destroyed by serum cholinesterase.

The hazards of relaxants are more related to the paralysis that they produce than to any individual properties. However, since they are so widely employed in anaesthesia, each will receive a brief introduction.

## 13.1  Competitive Blockers

Competitive blockers include tubocurarine chloride (Tubarine), gallamine triethiodide (Flaxedil), alcuronium chloride or diallylnortoxiferine (Alloferin), pancuronium bromide (Pavulon) and the recently introduced fazadinium (Fazadon).

### 13.1.1 Tubocurarine

Opinions differ about the effects of curare on the cardiovascular system. Some consider it has ganglion blocking properties because occasionally it causes a fall in blood pressure. However, ganglion blockers also induce tachycardia, and as no change in pulse rate follows the administration of curare, this explanation seems unlikely. More probably the fall in blood pressure is related to histamine release. Curare also reduces the incidence of cardiac arrhythmias: the reason is uncertain but it may be due to a blocking action on autonomic afferent pathways or a direct action on the myocardium.

*Interaction with Anaesthetic Agents.* Halothane potentiates the muscle blocking action of all relaxants interfering with neuromuscular transmission by desensitisation of the postjunctional membrane. Ether has muscle relaxant properties brought about by depression of nervous conduction in the spinal cord rather than by any specific neuromuscular action.

### 13.1.2 Gallamine

Gallamine triethiodide (Flaxedil) behaves like curare but has a shorter action. It is excreted by the kidney and is said to cross the placental barrier, so that it is contra-indicated in renal disease or obstetrics. There is less circulatory disturbance, since there is no histamine release or ganglionic blockade. Tachycardia occurs immediately after injection owing to a vagal blocking effect, therefore pre-existing tachycardia conditions exaggerating sympathetic activity are contra-indications.

A small amount (40 mg) of gallamine is often added to thiopentone in order to reduce reflex muscular activity, coughing etc. in patients having short procedures such as check cystoscopies or haemorrhoid operations.

### 13.1.3 Alcuronium

Alcuronium chloride or diallylnortoxiferine (Alloferin) like gallamine, has a short duration of action. It does not pass the placental barrier, and can be used in obstetrics, for which its short action is very suitable. No tachycardia follows administration, but it is excreted by the kidneys and should be avoided in the presence of renal failure.

### 13.1.4 Pancuronium

Pancuronium bromide (Pavulon) is a steroid derivative. It decomposes if kept at room temperature and must be stored in a refrigerator. Its duration of action is similar to that of curare, but the end point of relaxation is much clearer. It is said to cause release of noradrenaline, but not sufficiently to cause cardiovascular changes. As 50% is excreted by the kidney and 25% by the liver, it is best avoided in failure of either.

### 13.1.5  Fazadinium

Fazadinium bromide (Fazadon) was introduced in 1975 as a rapid-acting non-depolarising relaxant. Its rapidity of action makes it a suitable alternative to suxamethonium, especially in the presence of a full stomach (see Sect. 25.3.2). It is readily reversible by neostigmine and its duration of action is at least 15 min.

A mild trachycardia occurs, which probably, as in the case of gallamine, arises from some blocking effect on vagal tone. Excretion is mainly by the kidney so caution is advised in the presence of renal failure, though there is an alternative route for excretion through the liver. No evidence of histamine release exists, although there are reports of a flare over the vein or an urticarial rash after injection. There is a higher incidence of such reactions in children when small wrist veins are used and at present it is best avoided for children.

Fazadinium is an alternative to suxamethonium in obstetric anaesthesia. All reports of its use in obstetrics so far have been satisfactory. There is no evidence of placental transfer at full term, although in the case of other non-depolarising agents, small quantities may cross the placental barrier in early pregnancy.

### 13.1.6  Reversal of Competitive Blockade

As it is impossible to predict with accuracy the length of any operation, or how much relaxant a particular patient will require, sometimes anaesthetists find themselves with a paralysed patient at the end of an operation. An antidote is available for reversal of the non-depolarising relaxants but not of depolarisers.

Neostigmine (Prostigmin), an anticholinesterase, reverses non-depolarising relaxants by allowing acetylcholine to accumulate in sufficient quantity to displace curare from the motor end-plate, thus reversing the paralysis. Neostigmine is not without hazards. Accumulation of acetylcholine produces a muscarinic effect at the vagal nerve endings of the heart causing a bradycardia which, untreated, can cause cardiac arrest. Injection of atropine either before or together with the neostigmine neutralises the muscarinic action. To be safe, some anaesthetists inject atropine before neostigmine. But is has been shown that when atropine and neostigmine are injected together heart rate increases (owing to the atropine) within 25 s, whilst the effect of neostigmine only reaches its peak after 1½ min. The proportions are usually 1 mg atropine to 2.5 mg neostigmine.

The use of neostigmine to reverse curare after abdominal surgery has been criticised because its cholinergic action increases peristalsis and could harm a recently sutured anastomosis of the large intestine and rectum, but the criticism has not been substantiated.

Return of normal breathing, with a pause after expiration, indicates successful reversal of curarisation by neostigmine. Signs of inadequate recovery include persistence of an inspiratory pause together with a 'tracheal tug', ineffective coughing on the endotracheal tube, and the presence, sometimes, of fidgety, jerky, uncoordinated movements, especially of the head and neck.


## 13.2 Depolarising Relaxants

Two depolarising relaxants are in clinical use: decamethonium iodide and suxamethonium chloride or bromide.

### 13.2.1 Decamethonium

Decamethonium iodide (Eulissin) is no longer manufactured in the United Kingdom, although it is available in North America and Australia, and produces muscle relaxation by a depolarising block lasting about 20 min. Although decamethonium is free from undesirable side-effects, depolarisation sometimes gives way after repeated doses to a non-depolarisation type of blockade, the so-called Phase II, which presents diagnostic difficulties. For this reason, decamethonium is only used for short procedures not exceeding 1-1½ h. The maximum safe dose to avoid the Phase II block is considered to be 10 mg.

### 13.2.2 Suxamethonium

Preparations of suxamethonium chloride (Scoline) are liquid in ampoules containing 100 mg. Suxamethonium bromide (Brevidil B) is prepared in 100-mg ampoules in powder form which is mixed with sterile water. It is more stable than suxamethonium chloride, which must be stored in a refrigerator to prevent decomposition. Brevidil B can be stored in warm climates without fear of deterioration. The outstanding feature of the suxamethonium preparations is their capacity to produce rapid complete muscle relaxation of short duration (3 min) for tracheal intubation, for endoscopic (larynx, bronchi and oesophagus) examinations, for ECT and for closing an abdomen at the end of a long abdominal operation. The price paid in the form of hazards concerns the cardiovascular, muscular, alimentary and cholinesterase systems.

*Cardiovascular System.* There are no cardiovascular hazards for normal patients after a single dose, except an occasional rise in blood pressure. Repeated injections are said to cause bradycardia, sometimes to the point of cardiac arrest, especially if the second dose is given about 5 min after the first. This may be due to some vagal disturbance, since atropine, ganglion blockers and non-depolarising relaxants prevent it. Suxamethonium releases potassium from muscle of injured, burnt and paraplegic patients and can cause cardiac arrhythmias.

*Muscular System.* Many patients complain of severe muscle pains ('as though run over by a bus') 24-48 h after receiving suxamethonium. The incidence is 50% higher in ambulant than in bed-ridden patients. The cause is obscure and bears no relation to the amount of muscle fasciculation observed. Younger patients suffer less than older. A small dose of a non-depolarising relaxant, 40 mg gallamine, given 4 min before suxamethonium, reduces the incidence of muscle pain but also reduces the effectiveness of the suxamethonium.

The contraction of the extra-ocular muscles during fasciculation produces temporary increase in intra-ocular pressure, a disadvantage in ophthalmic surgery, especially in patients with glaucoma or detached retina or during cataract surgery. However, pressure rapidly returns to normal as the action of the drug wears off, and the use of suxamethonium in ophthalmic surgery for intubation is acceptable but should never be repeated after incision of the cornea (see Sect. 38.2).

*Alimentary System.* A dangerous hazard of suxamethonium is projectile-like regurgitation of stomach contents from increased intragastric pressure during muscle fasciculation, if the stomach is full (see also Chap. 25). Although rare in well prepared patients, it is never safe to assume that all patients have an empty stomach. From time to time patients are anaesthetised unknowingly with a stomach full of indigested food or faecal vomit from unsuspected obstruction. If given suxamethonium, such patients will certainly regurgitate, and if (as is so common) the anaesthetist is inflating the lungs, fatal aspiration will occur. Bourne records a fatality, the author has knowledge of two others and escaped a third only because he does not inflate the patient's lungs after injecting suxamethonium.

A better practice is to give oxygen before administering suxamethonium, and having injected the suxamethonium to wait, with laryngoscope and tube in hand, for fasciculations to cease and then insert the tube. On the occasion referred to, the laryngoscope was already in the mouth when the stomach contents welled up, but it was possible to put the tube in quickly and, by suction, prevent what would otherwise have certainly been a fatal outcome. The regurgitation is due to a rise in intra-abdominal pressure (see Sect. 25.2).

*Cholinesterase System.* Sometimes the action of suxamethonium is prolonged ('Scoline apnoea'). This occurs if a lack of serum cholinesterase (formerly known as pseudocholinesterase) in the blood or the presence of abnormal serum cholinesterase prevents hydrolysis or destruction of suxamethonium.

Normal blood contains two cholinesterase enzymes—acetyl and serum cholinesterase. Acetyl cholinesterase is widely distributed in red blood cells, nervous and muscular tissue, in cholinergic synapses and at the myoneural junction, and hydrolyses acteylcholine, but is ineffective on suxamethonium. Serum cholinesterase is formed in the liver and, whilst having little or no action on acetylcholine, destroys suxamethonium. Although not active in stored blood, serum cholinesterase is well preserved in fresh frozen plasma, which effectively supplements the enzyme if low serum cholinesterase levels prolong action of suxamethonium: (a) following radiotherapy; (b) after contact with insecticides containing phosphorus; (c) in hyperpyrexia; (d) in cardiac failure; (e) in liver failure and uraemia; (f) in malnutrition and anaemias; (g) following treatment of malignant disease with cyclophosphamide and of glaucoma with echothiopate iodide eye-drops (both substances antagonising cholinesterase); (h) in late pregnancy and the puerperium; and last but not least, (i) as a familial inherited abnormality which affects approximately 1 in 3000 of the population. In view of the wide spectrum of deficiency, the initial dose of suxamethonium should never exceed 50 mg. Even then, a patient with a congenital absence of serum cholinesterase may not breathe for up to 3 h.

Any patient whose respiration does not return within 15 min of 50 mg suxamethonium should be considered to have abnormal serum cholinesterase and treated for 'Scoline apnoea' as follows:

1) Manual or mechnical ventilation, with nitrous oxide and oxygen, should be given to spare any distress of return of consciousness whilst paralysed.

2) As carbon dioxide always accumulates before starting ventilation, plasma $P_{CO_2}$ should be measured; a raised carbon dioxide level is evident from a bounding pulse and flushed skin. Ventilation through a soda lime canister restores the level to normal.

3) An intravenous drip of 2 units of fresh frozen plasma will provide sufficient cholinesterase to reverse paralysis.

Properly treated, patients always recover from 'Scoline apnoea'. The rule is *not* to wait too long for return of respiration, but to start mechanical ventilation quickly together with a drip of fresh frozen plasma.

The serum of any patient with prolonged apnoea (and of all blood relatives) should be examined subsequently for abnormal cholinesterase. If present, all concerned should be instructed to inform hospital staff should they require anaesthesia. Congenitally abnormal serum cholinesterase resists the inhibitory action of dibucaine (cinchocaine, Nupercaine) compared with normal serum cholinesterase. The percentage inhibition of dibucaine (the dibucaine number, or DN) when cholinesterase is normal, is 97%, but when it is abnormal it is always prolonged, in the region of 16%-20%.

High serum cholinesterase levels can occur in obese subjects and in presence of thyrotoxicosis, nephritis, mental depression, psoriasis and alcoholism. In such subjects, the action of suxamethonium is shorter than usual.

### 13.3  Prolonged Apnoea After Non-depolarising Relaxants

Prolonged apnoea occurs after non-depolarising as well as depolarising relaxants, and fatalities have been recorded; this is probably the result not of prolonged action but of interference with the metabolism of the relaxant.

Neostigmine-resistant curarisation was a not uncommon condition 20 years ago after major abdominal operations on poor-risk and badly prepared patients. The anaesthetic technique consisted of large doses of non-depolarising relaxants, with anaesthesia maintained by nitrous oxide and oxygen. Neostigmine in double dosage failed to restore full muscle power, the patients maintaining a 'tracheal tug' during recovery. Mortality was high and patients died in circulatory failure, not respiratory failure, 6-8 h after operation. Less is heard of this conditon today. Two explanations offer themselves for the reduced incidence. Firstly, the introduction of halothane in 1956 provided a way of anaesthetising elderly poor-risk patients with half the conventional dose of relaxant, which made reversal by neostigmine easier. In addition, in the sixties the introduction of intensive care units greatly improved the treatment of respiratory and circulatory failure. Facilities for blood gas and electrolyte estimations provided better guidelines for organisation of treatment.

### 13.3.1  Causes

Prolonged apnoea following relaxants almost certainly arises from inability to metabolise the relaxant and opiates received during the operation, for reasons related to a poor physical state before operation. Amongst these are:

1) *Poor perfusion.* Elderly subjects and those with infection and incipient circulatory failure are susceptible to non-depolarising relaxants, whose action is often much prolonged, so that half the conventional dosage is often sufficient. Repeated doses 'saturate' receptors, so that paralysis persists for several hours because of the inadequacy of peripheral blood flow.

2) *Body temperature.* Lowering body temperature increases paralysis from depolarising relaxants but does not occur after non-depolarising relaxants. These observations have little relevance in clinical practice, except possibly at the end of long abdominal or thoracic procedures or following infusions of cold blood, when a significant loss of heat may occur.

3) *Carbon dioxide and blood* pH. Carbon dioxide retention prolongs

the action of curare but has little effect on paralysis from gallamine or depolarising agents. This applies to acidotic states, in which pH and $P_{CO_2}$ estimations should be carried out and any abnormalities on the acid side treated with an infusion of sodium bicarbonate—100 mmol in half an hour.

4) *Deficient renal function.* Curare is excreted by liver and kidney but gallamine is excreted only by the kidney. Depression of renal function or the shut-down which occurs in shocked states before appearance of signs of peripheral circulatory failure could cause prolonged apnoea after gallamine as well as after curare when liver function is depressed.

5) *Antibiotics.* The neuromuscular blocking action of some antibiotics can interfere with reversal of muscle relaxants. Streptomycin, neomycin, polymyxin, colistin, viomycin and paramycin possess weak neuromuscular blocking effects when placed intraperitoneally, especially in weak and debilitated patients. A major exception is the penicillin group. Successful reversal often follows injection of neostigmine with calcium chloride 200-500 mg or 5-12 mmol.

6) *Other causes.* When a patient fails to start breathing after anaesthesia, some of the more obvious causes other than relaxants should be eliminated before assuming that prolonged action or neostigmine resistance is present. Patients may not breathe because of central respiratory depression by opiates or a low plasma carbon dioxide. Return of respiration in these circumstances may follow intravenous injection of an analeptic such as nikethamide, vanillic acid or naloxone. Failure to respond eliminates these conditions.

Depression of the Hering-Breuer reflex and reflex laryngeal apnoea are also causes of absence of breathing. This is an ill-defined, poorly understood but harmless group. Sometimes patients with an endotracheal tube in place are reluctant to breathe at the end of long operations. Movement of the tube by deflating the cuff often provides the required stimulus for breathing. Possibly the trachea develops tolerance to the presence of the tube whilst the stretch receptors in the lungs themselves are depressed following interference with their control during artificial respiration, especially under halothane.

## 13.3.2 Treatment

When one has excluded the more obvious causes, mechanical ventilation should start immediately. Estimation of electrolyte and acid-base balance should be made and any abnormalities corrected.

The type of block should next be determined using a nerve stimulator (see Sect. 13.4 below). If the results indicate a depolarising type of paralysis, blood cholinesterase should be estimated and an infusion of fresh frozen plasma set up. If on the other hand a non-polarising or competitive blockade is present the patient should receive further injection of neostigmine and atropine.

**13.4   Nerve Stimulator**

The nerve stimulator is a small flat box, small enough to be held in the palm of the hand, containing a battery. Two electrodes project from the end to apply to the nerve to be tested. Nerve stimulators are used to determine whether a partially paralysed patient has a non-depolarising or depolarising type of block. Stimuli made through a switch are of two kinds: (a) single (twitch) 1-10 per second and (b) 'tetanic' 10-15 per second. Stimulation in the presence of non-depolarising block, after successive stimuli, reveals reduction of response, known as 'fade'. Following a volley of tetanic stimuli a single twitch stimulus produces an increased response, i.e. post-tetanic facilitation. A similar result follows administration of an anticholinesterase drug—neostigmine.

In depolarising block, single (twitch) stimulation or tetanic stimulation is characterised by well maintained response with no suggestion of fade.

Occasionally a patient, partially recovered from a depolarising block-ade, shows electrical responses characteristic of non-depolarising agents. This changed situation is responsive to anticholinesterase drugs. Thus, if recovery from a depolarising agent is slow, a nerve stimulator can demonstrate whether dual block has occurred or whether the patient has abnormal cholinesterase—knowledge vital to successful treatment.

# 14 Endotracheal Intubation

The passage of a tube into the trachea, whether through the nose or the mouth, is known as intubation, and probably presents more hazards than any other single anaesthetic procedure. It was originally introduced to facilitate surgery of the head and neck, and in particular, plastic surgery on soldiers injured in World War I. Subsequently the indications expanded to include, first, thoracic surgery following the development of controlled respiration with cyclopropane and carbon dioxide absorption, and later spread to abdominal surgery in order to provide adequate ventilation for patients paralysed by muscle relaxants.

In recent years intubation has become the rule rather than the exception and is often performed for any operation which is likely to last more than half an hour, on the grounds that it provides a safer airway. There are some signs that the pendulum is swinging the other way since the rediscovery that inhalational agents such as halothane, methoxy-flurane and enflurane can provide satisfactory relaxation for pelvic surgery with no need to intubate, since the head-down position prevents any danger of aspiration or secretions into the lungs.

The hazards of intubation can be subdivided into those associated with the equipment, those arising from anatomical abnormalities, and those arising during the performance of intubation and the subsequent operation.

## 14.1 Equipment

### 14.1.1 Laryngoscopes
Before inducing anaesthesia with the intention of passing an endotracheal

tube, a check of equipment is most necessary. The light source on the laryngoscope must be seen to be in working order and of sufficient brilliance. As batteries age, the light dims perceptibly and hinders recognition of landmarks in the pharynx and around the laryngeal aperture. Before use it is advisable to extend the blade forcibly to ensure the light will not go out owing to a faulty contact or loose bulb just as the larynx is exposed. Tightening the bulb should correct such a defect. If it fails to do so the instrument should be changed.

### 14.1.2  Endotracheal Tubes

The care of endotracheal tubes has improved immensely in recent years. Sterilisation is achieved either by autoclave (but not more than six times) or heating to 75°C for 10 min (pasteurisation), sufficient to destroy pathogenic organisms. Gamma rays are also used for sterilisation. Repeated heat sterilisation causes deterioration of rubber so that tube and cuffs become soft and liable to kinking.

Tubes should always be tested for kinking before use. If the two ends of the tube cannot be approximated without a kink forming, the tube should be destroyed because kinking of the tubes on movement of the head and neck or after 'bucking' can cause total obstruction to breathing.

The length of the tube is relevant; if the tube is too long, it will pass into the right main bronchus and cause collapse of the left lung; if too short, it can slip out of the larynx on movement of the head and finish up in the oesophagus. When the nasal route is used, the length should be twice the distance from the lobe of the ear to the nose. For oral use, 7.5 cm shorter.

The Oxford and nylon-reinforced tubes are a form of insurance against kinking. The Oxford tube is an inverted L-shaped tube, bent to conform to the curve over the tongue between mouth and pharynx. Although the diameter is constant the thickness of the part in the mouth and pharynx is twice that of the distal end, and for this reason it will not kink.

Nylon-reinforced tubes are made of plastic material into which a spiral of nylon has been incorporated, making kinking impossible. The tubes are straight when not in use, and for insertion a malleable metal introducer is needed. This should always be lubricated before use to prevent difficulty in withdrawal after successful intubation.

### 14.1.3  Endotracheal Connectors

The tube is connected to the anaesthetic apparatus via a metal angled endotracheal connector, whose other end connects with a small-diameter corrugated rubber tube known as the catheter mount, which is inserted into the gas outflow. Care should be taken that the metal connector fits firmly into the end of the tube; this is best assured by choosing a ribbed connector. Smooth connectors (e.g. the Magill pattern) can become detached from the tube, which is dangerous because if the connector is separated, the tube can disappear down into the pharynx or even into the trachea, posing problems of retrieval. Also a ventilator may appear to function normally although the patient, if paralysed, is receiving no anaesthetic, oxygen or air. If breathing is spontaneous or if the anaesthetist is inflating the lungs by hand, the defect is immediately evident.

Metal connectors need careful cleaning after use, for they can become obstructed with dried secretion or blood clot (there is even a record of obstruction by a dead cockroach!). Some connectors, e.g. the Cobb, have a removable rubber cap to allow suction down the tube during anaesthesia. Care should be taken to see that the cap fits firmly and is not perished.

## 14.2 Anatomical Abnormalities

Intubation, whether by the 'direct' oral or 'indirect' nasal method, depends for its success on the correct position of the head and neck. The cervical spine should be in full flexion and the head extended on the occipito-atlantal joint. This position is best obtained by flexion of the head on a firm pillow (plastic-filled pillows are useless as they do not fold when bunched up) followed by firm extension of the skull itself. It is necessary for the pillow to be firm so that maximum flexion of the cervical spine can be obtained. The object of this procedure is to bring as far as possible the mouth, pharynx and vocal cords into a straight line. Even when all these manoeuvres are carried out with care, difficulties can occur in about 10% of patients, in whom exposure of the larynx presents difficulties because of anatomical abnormalities.

### 14.2.1 Short Neck

The commonest difficulty is experienced with patients with a short, muscular ('bull') neck and a full set of incisor teeth. Flexion of the cervical vertebrae in such subjects is very limited, so that extension of the neck fails to bring the plane of the mouth even near that of the pharynx and larynx. The presence of a receding chin, usually with a short neck, only increases this difficulty, because there is an increase in the distance between the symphysis mentis and the lower alveolar margins, so that the lower jaw has to be depressed more than usual in order to visualise the larynx.

### 14.2.2 Teeth

Protruding upper teeth ('rabbit teeth') of themselves create difficulty because the blade of the laryngoscope is pushed too far forwards and thus cannot be levered sufficiently to expose the larynx. This condition is only made worse by a commonly associated high arched palate and long narrow mouth.

The presence of capped, filled or carious incisor teeth which cannot sustain the pressure of the laryngoscope blade mean that a lateral approach, using perhaps an eye tooth as a fulcrum, has to be attempted. Irregular dentition also presents problems, for if incisors are absent but the canine tooth remains, it often obstructs the passage of the tube.

### 14.2.3 Arthritic Changes

Finally, arthritic changes in the jaw or vertebrae of the neck, which limit movement, present difficulties which sometimes cannot be overcome even by experts and, as a last resort, tracheostomy may be necessary.

## 14.3 Hazards During Intubation

Damage to teeth and abrasion of lips and gums should not occur if teeth are checked beforehand and the laryngoscope manipulated with gentleness and care. If during intubation a tooth is loosened, provided that it is not actually falling out, it is better left in place and a dental opinion sought as soon as possible, as it should be following any dental complication, however trivial. Should a tooth be dislodged, every care must be taken to prevent it falling into the pharynx and thus into the trachea itself.

Trauma to the anterior fauces is sometimes not easy to avoid when conditions are difficult. It is remarkable how little discomfort this causes afterwards to patients. The vocal cords also suffer, especially when attempts are made to pass a tube in the presence of inadequate relaxation. Public speakers and singers need special care because there are on record cases where the voice has altered for some considerable time after the passage of an endotracheal tube. The larynx of young children and neonates is particularly delicate and liable to traumatic oedema following repeated unsuccessful attempts at intubation under inadequate anaesthesia (see also Sect. 36.6).

The presence of a large tube for a long period is another cause of damage. Granuloma of the cords themselves has been reported, but only rarely. However, hoarseness and sore throat sometimes occur after anaesthesia when no tube has been passed, but the incidence is higher following intubation. It is possible that coughing, and straining on the tube when it is in position, are contributory factors. Sore throat usually subsides in 24-48 h. Aspirin gargle will provide relief. Hoarseness should be treated by aromatic steam inhalation, e.g. tincture of benzoin in boiling water.

Nasal intubation, i.e. the passage of a tube into the larynx through the nose, presents additional hazards. Indications include any surgery—dental, ENT or plastic—on the mouth and pharynx. Resort to nasal intubation may also be necessary when for anatomical or other reasons it is not possible to visualise the larynx. Sometimes 'blind' intubation is attempted (for details, see standard textbooks); otherwise a laryngoscope and the Magill forceps are used to feed the tube into the larynx itself. Whatever method is used, the commonest and most difficult hazard is nasal haemorrhage. This can be considerably reduced by spraying the nose with 5% cocaine or some other vasoconstrictor such as phenylephrine about 20 min before passage of the tube. It is useless to spray the nose and pass the tube within a few minutes because the constricting action will not have had time to take its full effect. If bleeding does occur, the head should be lowered and suction performed, preferably with a soft rubber catheter, through the nose. Further attempts to intubate should not take place until the bleeding is under control. A tube slightly larger than the nasal entry, once in position, reduces bleeding by pressure.

An unusual complication of blind intubation is entrance and perforation of the pharyngeal pouch, which only becomes evident some weeks later as an abscess appearing in the neck from the posterior mediastinum.

The best way of avoiding most of the hazards mentioned so far is to ensure complete relaxation of the jaw muscles. This explains the popularity of suxamethonium, which provides total flaccidity within a few seconds of administration.

## 14.4  Hazards After Intubation

The most dangerous hazard following intubation is difficulty in inflating, or inability to inflate, the lungs, with associated persistent cyanosis of the patient. The temptation to blame the patient and diagnose 'bronchospasm' must be firmly resisted until all other technical reasons have been eliminated; these are:

1) Unexpected failure of the oxygen supply or even faulty connection of gas input

2) Kinking of a soft endotracheal tube

3) Over-inflation of a weak cuff, which has herniated over the end of the tube and blocked it

4) Blockage of the tube with foreign material, inspissated blood, etc.

5) Last but not least, *when the tube is in the oesophagus*; this occurs more frequently than many would believe.

The first action when faced with inability to inflate the lungs is to check the tube for kinking, either by feeling with a finger or by direct vision with a laryngoscope.

If no kink is found, then remove the connection to the machine, release the inflated cuff and blow down the tube. Failure to force air down the tube means an obstruction in the tube. If air goes down and does not return with recoil of the lungs, then the tube is in the oesophagus. It should be removed immediately and the lungs inflated with oxygen. Routine auscultation of the chest is the only certain way of confirming that a tube is in the right place. Observation can be misleading; rhythmic distension of the stomach with air through a tube in the oesophagus can give a false impression of chest movement and even wheezing sounds encourage diagnosis of bronchospasm. Distension of the stomach is transferred to the diaphragm thus encouraging sufficient movement to allow some gaseous exchange in the lungs, but not enough to maintain life. There is record of a stomach being perforated by inflation of oxygen through a tube in the oesophagus. Whenever difficulty is experienced during intubation, auscultation of the chest is the only sure way of making sure the tube is in the lungs.

### 14.5  Failure to Intubate

Apart from patients with fixed cervical spine or ankylosed jaws in whom difficulties in intubation can be anticipated, every so often one comes across a patient whose larynx cannot be visualised. Usually there is a combination of short neck, receding jaw and prominent backward-slanting incisor teeth.

No one likes to admit defeat, but after half a dozen attempts, which must always include passage of a nasal tube, a pause is advisable to review the position and consider whether it would be possible to carry on under inhalational anaesthetic without a tube. Apart from ENT, maxillo-facial, dental and transthoracic procedures, satisfactory operating conditions can be provided by inhalational techniques for most surgical procedures, including upper abdominal surgery.

Too vigorous instrumentation around the larynx during attempted intubation can result in haemorrhage and mucous secretion which make visualisation even more difficult and may lead to intractable laryngo-spasm when the effects of the relaxant wear off. The author has knowledge of two cardiac arrests (one fatal) in recent years, occurring during repeated attempts at intubation for lower abdominal procedures which could have been safely carried out under 2% halothane and oxygen.

If the operation cannot be carried out without a tube and there is no urgency, a postponement would be prudent to allow a planned approach at the next session, at which one of the following methods could be tried:

1) A thin gum elastic bougie or bent copper stylet can sometimes be passed through the larynx, after which the tube can be passed over it into the larynx itself and the bougie or copper stylet removed.

2) The reverse process has also been reported: an intracath or similar device is introduced through the cricothyroid membrane and passed

upwards into the mouth, from which it can be withdrawn and the tube threaded over the catheter and guided into the larynx. The catheter can then be withdrawn through the cricothyroid membrane.

3) A flexible fibre-optic laryngoscope can be passed through the nose or mouth, by means of which the pharynx and laryngeal aperture can be seen and the tube guided forward into the larynx. This procedure sounds simple but it is extremely difficult and it is not recommended for beginners. Considerable experience with a fibre-optic laryngoscope is necessary for any chance of success.

# 15 Positioning Patients for Surgery

Since anaesthetised patients feel no pain and cannot move, responsibility devolves on anaesthetists to ensure no harm ensues during operation, especially when the procedure requires unusual positions on the operating table. In addition to pressure on nerves, positions can embarrass respiration, they can be accompanied by changes in blood pressure, and they can cause venous obstruction. The following positions are in everyday use:

1) Supine
2) Prone
3) Lithotomy
4) Trendelenburg
5) Lateral

## 15.1 Supine

For most operations, patients are in the supine position (lying on the back). Stretching of the ulnar nerve may follow extreme flexion of arms on the chest for any length of time and they are better placed at the side or, for access to an intravenous infusion, one arm can be placed on an arm-board at an angle of 45°-50° to the trunk to avoid stretching the brachial plexus.

In most hospitals, plastic J-shaped splints are available to retain the arms by the side to prevent them slipping over the side of the operating table and damaging radial or ulnar nerves. Even arm-boards have hazards for, if too long, they pass under the patient to the opposite side and can cause pressure damage to the ulnar nerve of the other arm. The legs should not be crossed. A pillow or soft rubber roll should be placed under the Achilles tendon to raise the legs slightly and take pressure off the calf, to discourage thrombosis formation.

In the supine position the use of the gall bladder bridge can easily obstruct venous return from the abdomen and other dependent parts by kinking the inferior vena cava, producing rapid reduction of blood pressure. Effects are more severe after subdural or epidural block in which muscle relaxation is complete and sympathetic blockade has already produced fall in blood pressure.

## 15.2 Prone

In the prone position, patients lie face down. Before moving to this position, two pillows or soft rolls should be put on the operating table so that the pelvis rests on one and the chest on the other, to allow unhindered diaphragm movement and prevent congestion of abdominal veins, which can cause copious haemorrhage especially during laminectomy. The arms, as in the supine position, are better placed at the side, although often they are flexed—elbows out and hands under the head, a position sometimes adopted for sunbathing—which can be dangerous because stretching or pressure of the ulnar nerve can occur.

The physical act of turning patients needs great care. At least three people should be available. Anaesthetists should adopt a supervisory role and take no part in the turning other than ensuring that the head moves with the patient's trunk, that there is no stretching of the neck or damage to the cervical vertebrae, and that the endotracheal tube does not become dislodged. It is advisable to paralyse the patient before turning, otherwise coughing and spasm on the endotracheal tube is almost certain to occur and may cause kinking unless a nylon-reinforced tube has been used.

Damage to the cornea is particularly likely to occur in this position as the eyes may come into contact with pillows, and covering the patient's eyes before turning is a wise precaution. Indeed, pressure on the eye itself has caused retinal artery occlusion and blindness in one eye.

## 15.3 Lithotomy

In the lithotomy position the patient lies supine but the legs are raised on either side and the feet supported in slings attached to vertical metal poles. The position is used for all gynaecological and rectal operations as well as several urological procedures.

The chief hazard is pressure on calf muscles, predisposing to venous obstruction and thrombosis, and on the peroneal (or external popliteal) nerve, causing foot drop. This is particularly probable if the knees are placed inside the vertical metal supports. Diathermy burns from contact with the metal supports can occur, unless contact is prevented by cotton wool pads to separate the limbs from the metal.

### 15.4  Trendelenburg

The head-down position (Trendelenburg) for pelvic surgery probably holds more hazards than any other position, not least if the patient slides off the table. Such accidents are prevented by:

1) Shoulder supports. Unless carefully positioned laterally so that the acromion process takes the weight of the patient, there is risk of brachial plexus lesions from pressure.

2) A clove hitch round the ankles. This carries risk of pressure sores and venous obstruction and should not be used.

3) Use of a corrugated mattress. This is the safest and most effective method and a corrugated mattress should be standard equipment in every operating suite.

The steep head-down position can cause respiratory embarrassment in some patients. In young and slim patients there is little disturbance but in fat patients and those with large adbominal tumours serious reduction in tidal exchange and cyanosis may result, and in such cases it is better to paralyse with relaxants and maintain respiration by manual or mechanical ventilation.

Abduction of the arms to right angles or beyond can cause paralysis by stretching the brachial plexus. When it is necessary to have the arm away from the side of the patient, abduction should never exceed 90° and the forearm should be slightly flexed and pronated.

### 15.5  Lateral

The lateral position is often used for surgery of the kidney or chest, for abdominothoracic procedures and for transthoracic gastrectomy and oesophagectomy. The lower arm needs careful positioning to avoid venous obstruction, whilst the upper arm rests on a Carter-Braine holder with generous padding to avoid pressure on the ulnar nerve or contact with metal. Respiration is hindered to a certain extent in this position, and this is made worse if a bridge or inflated pillow is used to help access to a kidney. As already noted, bridges produce a fall in blood pressure from interference with venous return, but this can be countered by a little head-down tilt.

# 16 Maintenance of Anaesthesia

## 16.1 Awareness During Anaesthesia

Undoubtedly awareness during anaesthesia occurs more frequently today than in the past. There are several contributory factors, but one common to all is the widespread practice of paralysing patients for all major operations (irrespective of the need or otherwise for muscle relaxation) and maintenance of anaesthesia with nitrous oxide and a generous proportion (30% or more) of oxygen.

Under anaesthesia with spontaneous breathing, movement in response to pain accompanied by deepening of respiration, sometimes with stridor, draws attention to the imminence of returning consciousness. Paralysed patients are unable to respond to pain by movement or phonation; the only signs suggestive of insufficient anaesthesia are sweating (often marked following omission of atropine premedication), secretion of tears and a rise in systolic blood pressure.

Anaesthetists should bear in mind the possibility of return of consciousness in the following circumstances:

1) Induction with very short-acting intravenous agents, e.g. methohexitone, followed by a muscle relaxant, such as curare or pancuronium, which takes a short while to become effective. When a short-acting induction agent is used, a more powerful inhalational agent than nitrous oxide should be added to the inspired gases as soon as possible.

2) The omission of sedative premedication and of an intravenous induction agent, e.g. before caesarean section, have been shown to result in a high incidence of awareness during anaesthesia, with a degree of mental trauma which becomes evident in subsequent psychological disturbances.

3) Faults in mechanical ventilators and gas supplies, e.g. addition of air to anaesthetic gases due to leaking or discontinued connections. The nitrous oxide supply may fail unobserved, or the by-pass for anaesthetic gases may be left in the position for 'semi-open' techniques instead of diversion to the ventilator (East Radcliffe and Cape ventilators are particularly susceptible to this error).

## 16.2   Neurophysiology and Pharmacology of Awareness

The level of consciousness, i.e. awareness of self and environment, with all the gradations between deep sleep and the fully alert state, is dependent on the regulatory action of the subthalamic reticular formation over the cerebral cortex.

Alerting stimuli reach the reticular formation from collaterals which leave the classical sensory tracts as they pass up the brain stem on their way to the cerebral cortex. These collaterals synapse with ascending reticular neurones to form a secondary sensory pathway to the cortex.

All anaesthetics block conduction in the secondary sensory pathway, which is essential for consciousness, although conduction in the classical sensory pathways, the cerebral cortex, and the pyramidal tracts continues uninterrupted until the deeper planes are reached.

Pyramidal responses following sensory stimuli during anaesthesia have been measured in experimental animals. When the rate of pyramidal discharge exceeds a critical figure, movement of limbs takes place. In fact during light anaesthesia, cortical responses have been shown to be intensified, which gives rise to a suggestion that the reticular formation exerts an inhibitory as well as a regulatory action on the cerebral cortex. In this way it is possible to explain the struggling stage of ether (which has a powerful blocking action on the reticular formation) and post-operative restlessness from pain seen (particularly in children) after premedication with barbiturates, which in hypnotic doses depress arousal mechanisms only.

## 16.3   Spontaneous Movement Under Light Anaesthesia

All are familiar with spontaneous movement under light anaesthesia in response to painful stimuli, as well as the apocryphal remark of the surgeon to the anaesthetist, 'If the patient can stay awake, why can't you?'

While such movement is not necessarily indicative of return of consciousness, it is a strong signal for deepening anaesthesia and not (as is sometimes done) for administration of a muscle relaxant. In practice intravenous administration of an opiate succeeds in suppressing this movement, and the dose required, e.g. 25 mg pethidine, would have little effect on the consciousness of an anaesthetised subject.

It does appear however that its administration to a subject whose arousal has been partly suppressed by other drugs undoubtedly contributes to maintenance of unconsciousness. A possible explanation is that strong cortical stimulation, painful or otherwise, provides a feedback to the reticular formation through collaterals from the pyramidal tracts, evoking widespread sympathetic activity and noradrenergic response, major contributors to wakefulness.

## 16.4  Cortical and Subcortical Depression by Anaesthetics

Although all anaesthetics obtund the arousal response, the extent of suppression of the sensory cortex and motor response varies with each agent. Some, such as nitrous oxide and trichloroethylene, depress cortical receptiveness before consciousness, with resulting analgesia—a property exploited widely in midwifery.

Intravenous barbiturates, such as thiopentone, although they can in relatively low concentrations block the arousal mechanism, require much greater concentration to suppress response to pain. When used as the sole anaesthetic in the past, they caused serious cardiorespiratory depression and prolonged recovery.

The addition however of the analgesic effect of nitrous oxide in oxygen significantly reduced the dose of thiopentone required to maintain unconsciousness. Subsequently the practice of administering supplementary intravenous pethidine still further reduced the amount of thiopentone required for any operation.

Although producing significant analgesia, nitrous oxide on the other hand has a very feeble action on the arousal mechanism, particularly in robust subjects and alcoholics. In these patients consciousness is only lost when asphyxia contributes, and use of nitrous oxide for this purpose has virtually been abandoned.

Nevertheless the combination with a volatile agent such as halothane which has poor analgesic properties again reduces the overall concentration of this agent to maintain surgical anaesthesia.

## 16.5  Combinations of Tranquillisers and Opiates

The idea that combination of two agents, one depressing wakefulness and the other pain perception, can produce an overall depression of consciousness greater than either can produce alone even in increased dosage, is illustrated in various combinations of tranquillisers and opiates which are currently used in anaesthesia. The main tranquillisers in common use in anaesthesia are the phenothiazines, the butyrophenone derivative droperidol and the benzodiazepine derivative diazepam.

### 16.5.1  Phenothiazines and Opiates

The phenothiazine derivatives render the secondary sensory pathways more susceptible to the action of anaesthetics and hypnotics by reducing the strength of the stimulus entering the reticular formation by a deafferenting action, and hence prolong recovery unless the dosage of anaesthetic is reduced.

Intravenous injection of a potent agent such as chlorpromazine with an opiate to a patient who has already received heavy opiate pre-medication can result in loss of consciousness from simultaneous depression of the two sensory pathways as well as abolishing response to painful stimuli. This formed the basis of what was known some years ago as the 'lytic cocktail'. Prolonged recovery and transient hypotension made the technique unpopular.

If however 50 mg pethidine and chlorpromazine replaces conventional papaveretum and hyoscine premedication, an intravenous dose of the same quantities will result in a sleepy state in which response to pain stimuli remains. In these circumstances consciousness can be completely suppressed by administration of 80% nitrous oxide in oxygen with no further need for intravenous opiate supplements. Using this technique recovery is reasonably rapid, hypotension less pronounced and operative shock much reduced (see also Sect. 26.4.3).

Respiratory depression is never a problem with this technique as in neuroleptanalgesia because chlorpromazine effectively antagonises the respiratory depression of opiates, and will restore respiration following pethidine-induced apnoea.


### 16.5.2  Droperidol and Opiates

The butyrophenone derivative droperidol (Droleptan) combined with powerful short-acting synthetic opiates derived from pethidine, e.g. phenoperidine or fentanyl, was introduced as a less depressant alternative to the lytic cocktail, in a technique known as neuroleptanalgesia.

Droperidol is a tranquillising agent with a selective depressant effect on emotional response, one of the properties ascribed to the 'old' brain, also known as the rhinencephalon or limbic system. It has no direct action on the arousal mechanisms, and therefore has no hypnotic properties. When combined with phenoperidine or fentanyl, a state of partial analgesia and emotional indifference results. The dose of opiate required to obtain full immobility in the presence of painful stimuli is usually accompanied by unacceptable depression of respiration, which falls to 2-3 breaths per minute, so that assisted ventilation and abolition of consciousness become necessary. This usually takes the form of a sleep dose of a barbiturate, intubation after a muscle relaxant and mechanical ventilation with nitrous oxide and oxygen. Full loss of consciousness does follow, but adequate concentration of nitrous oxide and periodical supplements of opiate are essential. Severe respiratory depression may occur during recovery, requiring reversal with nalorphine or naloxone. Nevertheless, postoperative analgesia is often prolonged.

This technique has one serious disadvantage. Some patients become anxious and worried about the psychomotor paralysis they experience after droperidol. This affects them so much that many refuse a second exposure to the method. The incidence is difficult to assess, being minimised by those who advocate the technique and magnified by those who criticise it, but 7%-10% could be a fair figure.

### 16.5.3  Diazepam and Opiates

Diazepam has no anaesthetic or analgesic action but it does possess remarkable amnesic properties. Given intravenously in 5-10 mg dosage it provides complete amnesia for unpleasant endoscopic procedures such as gastroscopy which do not involve sensitive mucous membranes. Spontaneous movement occurring during such procedures is controlled by a small intravenous dose of opiates. Pentazocine hydrochloride (Fortral) is very popular because not being subject to the Dangerous Drugs Act regulations it is readily available at short notice.

Diazepam irritates small veins; painful thrombosis develops after 48 h in many instances and for this reason is seldom seen by whoever administered the diazepam in the first instance.

Some anaesthetists have used diazepam as an induction agent for administering a relaxant and passing an endotracheal tube. They rely presumably on its amnesic properties. It is difficult to justify such a practice when proper anaesthetic agents of equal safety are available.

## 16.6  Conclusion

Surgical anaesthesia is the result of a simultaneous depression of subcortical arousal mechanisms and the sensorimotor responses in the cerebral cortex. All anaesthetics except nitrous oxide depress both these mechanisms in varying degrees.

Tranquillisers and opiates can achieve the same object but to a limited degree. Suppression of response to pain stimuli and loss of consciousness result either in prolonged recovery, in the case of phenothiazines, or extreme respiratory depression, in the case of the butyrophenones. However, when they are given in reduced dosage and combined with nitrous oxide, abolition of consciousness and satisfactory surgical anaesthesia result.

# 17 Local Analgesia

Two types of hazard are associated with local analgesia: pharmacological hazards which, with the exception of cocaine, are common to all analgesics, and technical hazards associated with specific procedures.


## 17.1 Pharmacological Hazards

Apart from cocaine, all local analgesics are synthetic compounds. A benzene ring is a common chemical feature of all, and all possess actions on both central and peripheral nervous systems.

### 17.1.1  Cocaine

Cocaine, a naturally occurring derivative of the coca plant (the 'divine plant' of the Incas) differs from the synthetic compounds in several respects, particularly in its central nervous action, and justifies separate attention. Karl Koller in 1884 drew attention to the local analgesic properties of cocaine. An American surgeon, Halstead, and a colleague working in Paris undertook personal experimentation into its anaesthetic properties and tragically discovered its most dangerous hazard—addiction. Halstead was cured but his colleague died. Halstead's personality changed completely from one of cheerful extroversion to that of a morose introvert.

Cocaine is never used for infiltration anaesthesia because of its addictive properties; only preparations with a surface action are available, in solutions of 2%, 5% or 10% in water as well as a 20% solution in the form of a paste.

*Toxic Effects.* Cocaine has a strong sympathomimetic action and enhances the effects of any sympathetic stimulation, e.g. that of injected adrenaline or of circulating adrenaline due to apprehension. The association of cocaine with subsequent injection of local analgesic solutions containing adrenaline is highly dangerous; cardiac arrhythmias, ventricular fibrillation and cardiac arrest have occurred. Cocaine should always be used alone.

*Central Action.* Cocaine in small amounts causes excitement and euphoria (hence its addictiveness) but high dosage results in unconsciousness and convulsions. The maximum dose of cocaine is 16 mg. Absorption of 10% concentrations is slower than that of 5% of 2%, since the vasoconstriction accompanying the higher concentration delays absorption.

*Indications.* Cocaine is used exclusively to anaesthetise surface membranes of the eye, nose and upper respiratory tract, including the trachea. In the eye, pupillary dilatation increases intraocular pressure and should be avoided in sufferers from glaucoma. Repeated applications to the eye can cause clouding and ulceration of the cornea; cocaine is therefore not used, since alternatives are available which dilate the pupil and produce vasoconstriction and local analgesia.

Cocaine spray constricts the nasal mucous membrane and reduces bleeding during the passage of nasal endotracheal tubes. The 20% cocaine paste is applied intranasally to reduce bleeding during intranasal operations.

Cocaine sprays are used to produce local analgesia in the throat before endoscopy without general anaesthesia. Care must be taken that the nozzle of the spray is secure, since it can become detached and pass into the bronchi. Injection of 2 ml of 10% cocaine through the cricothyroid membrane will provide good local analgesia of trachea and bronchi before bronchoscopy.

Plastic and ENT surgeons often inject local analgesics containing adrenaline or saline solutions containing adrenaline to reduce bleeding in operations on the head, neck and nose. In these circumstances, cocaine sprays and nasal paste must never be used.

### 17.1.2 Synthetic Local Analgesics

Table 1 gives basic information on the use of common local analgesics. Length of action varies from just under 1 h for procaine to up to 4 h for cinchocaine.

*Central Action.* Local analgesics depress the central nervous system as well as peripheral nerves. The first effect of overdose is drowsiness and insensitivity to pain (see particularly lignocaine), which anaesthetists in poorer countries exploit to provide surgical anaesthesia, supplemented with opiates and relaxants. Intravenous infusion of local analgesics has been used to relieve postoperative pain, but the method has now been replaced by continuous epidural block.

Early indications of overdose are restlessness and spontaneous movements of the limbs. Unless administration is stopped and an antidote given, progress to convulsions, coma and respiratory failure will occur.

Thiopentone or diazepam, given intravenously, is an effective antidote and a syringe filled ready for use should always be available if a local block requires large amounts of solution, e.g. abdominal field block or paravertebral block, or local block for thoracoplasty.

*Use of Adrenaline.* All synthetic local analgesics are vasodilators, hence absorption is rapid. To avoid this and reduce bleeding, adrenaline 1:1000 is added to the solution to bring dilution to not less than 1:80000, for dental work, or 1:200000 for local infiltration of large amounts (see Table 1). Adrenaline is unstable, and is only added at the last moment to the local analgesic. To avoid accidental overdose or ventricular fibrillation, anaesthetists should insist on checking the ampoule. Vacuum cartridges for ENT and dental surgery are exceptions.

*Cardiovascular Effects.* Complaints of palpitations, flushing and fullness in the head after injection of local analgesic solutions are almost always the result of adrenaline and subside especially with momentary suspension of surgical activity.

Whilst true allergic sensitivity is doubtful, the sight of a syringe and needle can produce faintness and vasovagal attacks. Premedication with tranquillisers or barbiturates reduces the incidence of these side-effects.

Local analgesics also have a direct action on the heart. Procainamide causes heart block of quinidine-like nature and lignocaine has anti-arrhythmic properties. The electrocardiogram of procainamide shows a wide QRS complex, which gives rise to extrasystoles and fibrillation. An unexplained vagolytic action may cause tachycardia. For this reason, procainamide has been replaced by lignocaine, which does

**Table 1.** Local analgesics in everyday use.

| | Cocaine | Procaine (Novocain) | Lignocaine (Xylocaine) | Bupivacaine (Marcain) | Prilocaine (Citanest) | Cinchocaine (Nupercaine) |
|---|---|---|---|---|---|---|
| Surface application | 2%-10% Nasal paste (20%-25%) | No | 4% | No | 4% | 1-mg lozenges |
| Local infiltration | Never | 0.5%-1% Solution | 0.25%-0.5% | 0.25% | 0.5%-1.0% | Not used |
| Nerve blocks | Never | 1%-2% | 1%-1.5% | 0.5% | Brachial plexus 1% | Not used |
| Adrenaline for vasoconstriction and slow absorption | Never | 1:100 000 to 1:200 000 | 1:100 000 to 1:200 000 | 1:100 000 to 1:200 000 | Dental 4% 1:300 000 | No |
| Epidural, caudal or spinal | Never | 5% without adrenaline | Epidural or caudal 1.5% with adrenaline 5 µg/ml Spinal 5% | Epidural or caudal 0.5% | Epidural 1.5% Spinal 'heavy' 5% in 5% glucose | 'Heavy' Nupercaine 0.5% in 6% glucose, 2-3 ml 'Light' Nupercaine 1:1500 in 0.5% saline, 12-20 ml |
| Maximum dose | 2 ml 10% 4 ml 5% 200 mg | 0.5-0.8 g 500 ml 0.5% 250 ml 1% 125 ml 2% | 0.5 g 50 ml 0.5% 100 ml 0.25% with adrenaline | 0.15 g 30 ml 0.5% 60 ml 0.25% with adrenaline | 400 mg 600 mg with adrenaline | 3 ml 0.5% 20 ml 1:1500 |
| Duration | Up to 1 h | 30-45 min | 45-60 min | 1-1½ h | 1½-2 h | 2-3½ h |

not depress the heart, although it effectively controls irregularities of rhythm, especially after myocardial infarction. Since the optimum intravenous dose of lignocaine closely approximates the maximum tolerated dose, drowsiness and loss of consciousness may occur. Alternatively, after too small a dose, dysrhythmias will recur. Patients under treatment need constant attention over 24 h and should be cared for in an intensive care unit.

## 17.2  Types of Procedure—Nerve Blocks

Local analgesic procedures vary from local infiltration and blocking of individual nerves, to caudal, epidural or subdural blockade. One common hazard is inadvertent intravenous injection. There are two ways of avoiding this complication. During subcutaneous infiltration of local analgesic solutions, e.g. for thyroidectomy, the needle should be kept moving continuously back and forth, so that even if a vein is entered it passes through before any significant quantity of fluid can enter the circulation.

During performance of nerve blocks, on the other hand, the local analgesic is concentrated in a small area. Aspiration should be made immediately before injection: absence of blood aspirate indicates it is safe to proceed.

### 17.2.1  Orbital Block

During block of the long and short ciliary nerves within the muscle cone of the eye to produce analgesia and absence of movement, perforation of the blood vessels sometimes leads to haematoma formation with proptosis. Although appearing extensive, it usually subsides without very active treatment. Aspiration is inadvisable unless great tension exists. Simultaneous injection of hyaluronidase ensures rapid absorption of any haematoma.

### 17.2.2  Brachial Plexus Block

Anaesthesia of the brachial plexus follows injection of 30-40 ml of 1% lignocaine in 1:100000 adrenaline, either by the supraclavicular route onto the plexus as it passes over the neck of the first rib behind the subclavian artery or by the axillary approach on either side of the artery. Technical details can be found in any standard textbook or better still a monograph on local analgesic methods.

An obvious hazard common to both procedures is intra-arterial or intravenous injection. Aspiration before injection for this procedure is absolutely essential. Should the needle penetrate an artery, it should be withdrawn and continuous pressure applied (after completion of the block) for 10 min.

The supraclavicular approach has two main hazards: pneumothorax, in 4%-5% of patients, requiring intercostal drainage; and paralysis of the phrenic nerve with hemiparesis of the diaphragm and collapse of the base of the lung on that side.

Horner's syndrome (enophthalmos—dropping of the upper eyelid and dilatation of the pupil) may occur if the solution reaches the superior cervical ganglion. The nose also may become blocked on the same side owing to congestion, and there will be flushing of the skin and neck with absence of sweating, also on the same side.

The axillary approach lacks these hazards and is simpler to perform successfully, but the analgesia does not include the shoulder joint, for which this procedure is often used in reducing a dislocation. Analgesia is limited to the forearm, restricting the usefulness of this approach.

Occasional failure and pulmonary complications explain why brachial block is not employed more widely.

Retrograde intravenous lignocaine with a tourniquet is a useful and ingenious method of producing analgesia in the forearm and hand or ankle and foot. It was first described in 1908 but little used until the 1960s. It is popular in emergency and accident departments, being less time-consuming than local blocks. After placing an indwelling intravenous needle on the dorsum of the hand or foot, preceded by exsanguination of the limb by Esmarch bandage, a tourniquet cuff blocks the arterial supply and on removal of the Esmarch bandage 40 ml of 0.5% lignocaine is injected intravenously. Good analgesia follows, although the exsanguinating cuff can cause discomfort if applied too high.

It was thought that the blood level of lignocaine might reach toxic limits on release of the tourniquet, but estimation of lignocaine blood levels have not substantiated this, However, care should be taken not to exceed the prescribed limit when using the method for analgesia of the lower limb.

### 17.2.3   Intercostal Block

Pneumothorax may result. When the paravertebral approach is used, spread of the solution can cause sympathetic blockade. This can be avoided by injecting the solution in the intercostal angle under the rib.

### 17.2.4   Lumbar Sympathetic Block

Surgeons sometimes ask anaesthetists to carry out lumbar sympathetic block to assess what improvement in blood supply of arteriosclerotic limbs would follow a permanent lumbar sympathectomy. The existence of large blood vessels in this area make the hazards of arterial or intravenous injection very real.

Intrathecal or epidural injection may occur, as well as paralysis of the third lumbar nerve by retrograde spread of the solution. Aspiration before injection is essential and patients must be carefully watched for 20 min after the procedure to make sure intrathecal or epidural spread has not occurred.

### 17.2.5  Pudendal Block

About 80 ml of 0.5% lignocaine is required, which is near the upper limit of safety. The cervix does not become insensitive, thus intra-uterine manipulations are precluded. Its main use is to allow painless episiotomy and subsequent repair.

### 17.2.6  Dental Blocks

Local analgesia is widely used in dental surgery. The strength of adrenaline is greater than that used elsewhere, but only a small amount (1-2 ml) of local analgesic is necessary to abolish pain. Care is needed to avoid intravenous injection when blocking the inferior dental nerve, for the high concentration of adrenaline carries a greater hazard than in other conditions.

## 17.3  Epidural Block

Epidural analgesia is produced by injection of local analgesic solutions in the space between the spinal cord with its coverings and the vertebral canal, where it reaches the nerve roots as they emerge through the intervertebral foramina. Relatively large quantities of fluid are necessary. The chief difficulty is making sure the injection is placed correctly.

The method was introduced after World War I and has achieved wide popularity in spite of the time taken to induce analgesia and in spite of an established failure rate. Painless childbirth under epidural analgesia has earned it widespread popularity among obstetricians and patients, wherever trained staff are available. As in other procedures requiring special training, a major hazard is inexperienced staff. There are many other hazards, some major and some minor, which the late Dr. Massey Dawkins, who pioneered the method, compiled and analysed some years ago.

Hazards of epidural analgesia can be divided into those associated with single injections into the extradural space of the thoracic and lumbar region, those associated with introduction of indwelling catheters and those associated with caudal blocks.

### 17.3.1  Single Injections

*Dural Tap.* The incidence of dural tap varies between 0.5% and 7.5% and is related to the method adopted to identify the epidural space. Resistance techniques, the simplest and commonest in use, have the highest incidence. Of the mechanical devices designed to facilitate recognition of the epidural space, a modification of the Brooks indicator, which requires a source of heat, gives the lowest incidence of dural tap. Odom's indicator is amongst the least reliable of these devices.

Failure to recognise a dural tap constitutes a major hazard, because injection of the full amount of solution necessary for an extradural block will result in a total spinal, i.e. paralysis of the entire spinal cord. Should such a catastrophe occur, artificial ventilation should be undertaken, preferably with a mechanical ventilator, and an intravenous infusion of 1:250 000 adrenaline in normal saline started, combined with a head-down tilt to counteract the fall in blood pressure from total sympathetic paralysis. After a dural tap has occurred, the needle should be withdrawn and another space utilised.

Headache is an unwelcome complication of dural tap. Injection of 30 ml normal saline into the space concerned has been recommended. Patients should lie flat for 24 h. Drugs such as diazepam or chlorpromazine given orally and conventional analgesics usually give relief. Attempts to relieve headache by cortisone injection of the space concerned should be avoided at all costs.

*Puncture of a Blood Vessel.* This is more common than dural puncture (2.8%). Usually it is evident if blood issues from the needle or enters the catheter. The space must be immediately abandoned to avoid possible intravenous injection of local analgesic.

*Epidural Haematoma.* After epidural puncture haematoma can be large enough to compress nerve roots, with sufficiently severe sciatic pain to require laminectomy.

*Convulsions.* Overdose or idiosyncrasy to the drug employed can cause convulsions. They are more common after amethocaine (0.7%), whose use has been largely abandoned in favour of lignocaine.

*Massive Epidural.* What is known as a massive epidural sometimes occurs about 20 min after an apparently normal block. Respiration fails slowly and pupils dilate, but blood pressure remains stable. Although cyanosis is absent, possibly because a certain amount of air moves in and out of the lungs with cardiac pulsations, prudence dictates the need for mechanical ventilation, if only to avoid the accumulation of carbon dioxide. If 2% lignocaine was the analgesic used, the patient will usualy wake *suddenly* after 1¼ h and equally suddenly resume normal breathing. These two observations distinguish this condition from a total spinal. Following total spinal, blood pressure becomes unrecordable and respiration stops completely, accompanied by cyanosis. Recovery of respiration after total spinal, far from being sudden, takes at least 30 min after the appearance of return of muscle activity, usually in the form of a tracheal tug.

The incidence of this bizarre complication is between 0.1% and 0.3%. No explanation is forthcoming at present, although transudation of solution across the dura mater from the extradural space is a possibility.

*Hypotension.* The point at which hypotension becomes a complication is a matter of individual opinion. Evidence accumulates yearly that falls in blood pressure consequent on reduction in vasomotor tone or active tension resulting in a lowering of critical closing pressure are not harmful, because perfusion is maintained (see Sect. 18.1). In spite of this, it should be routine to have an intravenous infusion running before starting induction of epidural analgesia. Although patients under spinal analgesia tolerate fall in blood pressure with no ill effect, induction of epidural analgesia with a solution containing adrenaline can be dangerous. Adrenaline induces *local* vasoconstriction increasing critical closing pressure locally, well above that in the rest of the circulation, where sympathetic paralysis has reduced vasomotor tone and critical closing pressure. A fall in blood pressure to 10.7 kPa compromises flow in the constricted area with high critical closing pressure, producing local damage to neighbouring nervous tissue. This is a possible explanation for reports of paraplegia following epidurals in which adrenaline was added to the local analgesic.

*Hypertension.* High blood pressure on recovery occurs rarely, usually in patients who were hypertensive beforehand.

*Backache.* After epidural analgesia backache occurs from time to time. The incidence is greater following the trauma to ligaments caused by a blunt needle.

### 17.3.2 Indwelling Catheters

After insertion into the epidural space, catheters will go in the direction the operator intends in only about 25% of patients. In over half, it just curls up at the point of entry, in 18% it forms a single loop, and in 6% it emerges through an intervertebral foramen. These figures are the result of X-ray control in nearly 300 patients and indicate the advisablility of inserting the needle at the *midpoint* of the segments which it is desired to anaesthetise and *initially* not to inject more than 5 ml of solution.

Failure of the catheter to enter the epidural space at the first attempt occurs in 4%, but often a second attempt is successful, bringing the failure rate down to the region of 2%.

Once the catheter is inserted, problems may arise in its connection to a syringe. Three possible courses are open, each having its own drawback:

1) To leave the Tuohy needle threaded on the catheter and connect its expanded end to the syringe. The catheter may kink as it leaves the side opening of the needle, as it may also at the junction with the expanded end.

2) Alternatively, one can remove the Tuohy needle, cut off the expanded end of the catheter and insert a hypodermic needle of sufficient size to give a tight fit. Besides decreasing the lumen, the needle point can perforate the wall and cause a leak.

3) A ureteric catheter adaptor can be connected to the cut end of the catheter, again narrowing the lumen, but avoiding the possibility of puncture.

The perfect method of connection is still awaited.

*Perforation of Dura by Catheter.* This is a particularly dangerous hazard, especially if a test dose of analgesic solution prior to insertion of the catheter indicates the Tuohy needle is in the correct place. In these circumstances total spinal can occur. A safer course of action is to delay the test injection until the catheter is in place.

*Broken Catheters.* Since broken catheters are sterile and not irritant, they cause no problems and should always be left alone.

*Site of Passage of Catheter.* Catheters pass more easily in the mid-thoracic region than the lumbar region and the rate of dural tap is reduced. In the thoracic region, approach is at an angle of 45° to avoid the overhanging thoracic spine and thus brings the side opening of the Tuohy needle opposite the middle of the epidural space. In the lumbar region, on the other hand, the needle enters at a right angle, making passage of the catheter much more difficult.

### 17.3.3 Caudal Block

Caudal block is produced by injection of a local analgesic solution into the sacral hiatus, where it comes into contact with the sacral nerves.

*Anatomical.* In 5% of patients the diameter of the sacral hiatus is less than 2 mm, causing uncertainty in where to insert the needle and failure to identify the hiatus in about 3% of patients. The dural sac ends, on average, 43 mm from the hiatus, but it can be as little as 19 mm. Dural puncture, however, is very rare (1.2%); accidental spinal occurred in only 0.1% of patients.

Malposition of the needle is more likely in fat patients. The commonest malposition is when the needle is posterior to the sacrum. If in doubt, injection of air from a syringe causes surgical emphysema, detectable by placing a hand over the sacrum. Rarely the needle passes forward and has twice entered the skull of the foetus with fatal results. When palpating the sacral hiatus in the lateral position, it should be remembered that the sacral crease lies 1 cm below the hiatus, owing to the effect of gravity.

*Sepsis* is a hazard because puncture in this area is adjacent to the rectum.

*Headache* is unknown as dural tap hardly ever occurs, but backache is fairly common at 7.6%, four times that following epidurals.

*Breakage of needle or catheter* is more common than after epidural, largely because most patients are restless, being in childbirth. Nevertheless accurate catheter placement (88%) is better than in epidurals and the forceps rate much lower (14% compared with 44%).

*Severe hypotension,* with blood pressure falling to below 10.7 kPa is commoner, surprisingly enough, after caudal block than after lumbar block. A possible explanation is the larger amount of analgesic drug used than for epidural.

### 17.3.4 Failure

Overall failure rate of caudal and epidural blocks is about 2%. Apart from inexperience the following are contributory factors:

1) Obesity making identification of anatomical landmarks impossible
2) Osteo-arthritis making penetration of calcified ligaments impossible
3) Repeated dural tap
4) Repeated puncture of a blood vessel
5) Injection in the wrong place, although extradural, or in insufficient quantity

### 17.3.5  Anticoagulant Therapy a Contra-indication

Anticoagulant therapy should be considered a contra-indication to use of epidural analgesia. Dawkins refers to two patients receiving anti-coagulants who developed extradural haematoma with compression of the cord, causing a permanent paralysis in one patient and paralysis with recovery after 10 months in the other.

## 17.4  Subdural Block

Subdural or 'spinal' analgesia is produced by placing the analgesic solution in direct contact with the spinal nerves by means of a fine needle passed through the theca. Less solution is required than for epidural analgesia and the method is more certain and precise, besides taking much less time to carry out.

The adoption of muscle relaxants in anaesthesia for abdominal surgery, together with litigation arising from allegations of negligence from patients paralysed following spinal analgesia, led to the almost complete disappearance of the method in Great Britain for many years. There has recently been a revival of interest.

Although hazards are few and seldom fatal, the consequences can be devastating. The hazards can be divided into several groups and arise from the following causes:

Faults in preparation of equipment and agents

Faults in personal preparation

Errors in choice of patients and their preparation

Errors in the performance of lumbar puncture

Choice of agent and dosage administered

Faults during administration

Complications following spinal analgesia

### 17.4.1  Preparation of Equipment

One serious complication of spinal analgesia, a subject of litigation, arose because all instruments were immersed in sterile water before use, after sterilisation by boiling. In that particular hospital the so-called sterile water came from a tank found to contain non-pathogenic Gram-negative water organisms. Although these organisms do not proliferate in peripheral tissues, they do proliferate in cerebrospinal fluid, which provides ideal culture conditions. Multiplication of these organisms caused irritation and chronic leptomeningitis with consequent paraplegia.

Such complications can be completely avoided by forbidding the use of sterile water in any form during performance of spinal analgesia and insistence on dry sterilisation of all equipment by heat or gamma ray. Gamma ray sterilised disposable packs containing needles and solutions are ideal.

### 17.4.2  Preparation of Agents

Some years ago, unexplained postspinal paraplegia gave rise to litigation. The defence alleged that the cause was contamination of a cracked ampoule containing the analgesic solution by spirit or other antiseptic solution in which it had been stored, and successfully demonstrated that contamination could occur in this way. Immersion of ampoules in antiseptics has now been abandoned. Ampoules of local analgesic solution are now included in the spinal pack or in separate containers sterilised by heat.

### 17.4.3  Personal Preparation

Preparation for induction of spinal analgesia should not differ from that before major surgery, i.e. scrub up and put on gowns, masks and sterile gloves. Such preparation may appear unnecessarily cautious until one recalls how devastating the consequences of infection are. Every effort must be made to avoid it.

### 17.4.4  Choice of Patients

Spinal analgesia should never be performed on dehydrated, hypo-volaemic or shocked patients. In such patients the ensuing sympathetic paralysis expands capacitance and reduces the effective circulating blood volume almost to the point of circulatory collapse. Spinal analgesia should only be undertaken after resuscitation by intravenous fluids.

### 17.4.5  Preparation of the Patient

The proximity of the puncture site (L 3-4) to the rectum is reason for rectal preparation after thorough cleansing, preferably in the bath, after bowel action. Skin preparation of the back, as for surgery, including shaving when necessary, should always by undertaken. The presence of infection of the skin of the back or of the rectum is a contra-indication to spinal analgesia.

### 17.4.6  Performance of Lumbar Puncture

The skin should be cleansed with antiseptic fluid and towels placed across the lower part of the back at the level of the iliac crests before performing lumbar puncture.

A 22 gauge needle is small but sufficiently rigid not to buckle on passage through the tough spinal ligaments. Subcutaneous injection of local analgesic at the site of puncture is optional and can obscure the intervertebral space. Most patients tolerate the passage of the spinal needle without complaint. After identifying the space between L3 and L4 and before attempting puncture, the needle should be held perpendicular to both vertical and transverse planes, and the needle inserted in the direction of the patient's umbilicus. If, after two or three attempts, no cerebrospinal fluid is obtainable, the space above or below should be tried. If attempts in all three spaces fail it is better to abandon the procedure. Common causes of failure are extensive osteo-arthritic change and scoliosis with rotation of vertebrae pulling the spinal canal out of line.

Damage to the cauda equina is a hazard of lumbar puncture. The cauda equina normally ends at the lower level of the first lumbar vertebra, but in a few patients it reaches the upper border of the second. If puncture is restricted to the spaces between the second and third, third and fourth, fourth and fifth lumbar vertebrae, no damage to the cauda equina is possible. The space between L3 and L4 can easily be identified by placing a hand along the tip of the iliac crest: a thumb placed horizontally will come to rest in the space between L3 and L4.

### 17.4.7  Choice of Agent and Dosage

Overdose is unlikely, provided not more than one ampoule of solution is used. Solutions in common use are hypobaric cinchocaine (Nupercaine; 1:1500) and three hyperbaric solutions: cinchocaine 1:200 in 6% dextrose, mepivacaine 4% in 9.5% dextrose, and prilocaine (Citanest) 5% in 5% glucose. So-called hypobaric solutions are said to rise in the theca, but evidence suggests displacement by volume injected takes place. If 20 ml is injected between L3 and L4, one can expect analgesia up to the nipple line. For most abdominal operations 12-14 mil is sufficient. Analgesia of a similar extent will be given by 2 ml heavy cinchocaine or lignocaine injected between L3 and L4.

### 17.4.8  Spread of Heavy Solutions

Heavy solutions obey the law of gravity and when injected with a patient on the side, the major part of action will be seen on the dependent side.

Head-down tilt after heavy spinal is often regarded as dangerous. Such fears are groundless since the solution is fixed by the nervous tissue within 15 s. After half a minute it is unlikely that any further spread will take place and there is no danger in tipping the patient into a head-down position.

### 17.4.9 Complications

As after epidurals, a drop in blood pressure follows induction of spinal analgesia. It is therefore customary to include an intravenous infusion whenever analgesia is above the umbilicus. Injection of a vasopressor such as ephedrine intramuscularly at the same time as induction of analgesia is also used to counter hypotension. The more widespread use of intravenous infusions during surgery has rendered this precaution unnecessary.

*Nausea and Vomiting.* An occasional distressing complication is nausea and vomiting. Traction on the mesentery, especially near the coeliac plexus, has been blamed, but nausea and vomiting may occur even before incision of the skin. It has been suggested that the cause is increase in central vagal tone following sympathetic paralysis, which is also evident in progressive slowing of pulse rate. Nausea and vomiting can be prevented by intravenous injection of up to 50 mg each of pethidine and promethazine immediately after induction of analgesia. Intravenous injection of 5-10 mg diazepam is an alternative.

*Spinal Headache.* Opinions differ about the cause of postspinal headache, which occurs in 5%-7% of patients. Leakage of cerebrospinal fluid through the puncture needle is a popular explanation, but the absence of headache when cerebrospinal fluid leaks elsewhere, for example following head injuries, casts doubt upon this suggestion. However, supporters of the leakage theory draw attention to figures which show that the incidence of headache varies directly with the size of the needle and thus the size of the hole made through the theca. Traumatic puncture could also cause headache from the irritation set up by the trauma to the dural sac and haematoma formation after puncture of one of the plentiful postspinal veins.

The use of fine sharp needles during lumbar puncture reduces the incidence of headache. However, the very fine needles should not be used by beginners, only by those who have considerable experience. A suitable size is 22 gauge, which is not associated with a high incidence of headache. Finer needles are difficult to handle and certainly should be avoided by beginners. All patients should lie flat for 24 h after lumbar puncture; this reduces the incidence of headache considerably.

Headache should be treated by enforced rest in the horizontal position with administration of oral analgesics and tranquillisers. Chlorpromazine has been reported to be particularly helpful in these conditions. If headache is severe, the chlorpromazine should be given intramuscularly in a dose of 50 mg. If leakage is thought to be the cause, considerable improvement has been claimed to follow subarachnoid injection of up to 30 ml normal saline, with the object of raising the cerebrospinal pressure and preventing leakage at the puncture site. It has even been suggested that a catheter should be placed in the epidural space through which a continuous infusion should be administered.

*Neurological Sequelae.* Mention has already been made of possible nerve damage by infection or damage to the cauda equina. From time to time, however, neurologists make allegations of neurological damage following spinal analgesia. Usually these reports concern patients referred to them with unexplained neurological disease who at some time *previously* have undergone spinal analgesia. The inference is either that non-specific damage occurred during lumbar puncture, or that the solutions used had an irritant effect. If a lumbar puncture is a cause, it is strange that similar damage has never been reported following diagnostic lumbar puncture by physicians.

It is also strange that neurological sequelae do not appear to follow the more bulky and equally irritant contrast solutions used in myelography.

It is generally agreed by anaesthetists who practise spinal analgesia that neurological complications can be ascribed either to a latent disease or to a disease that had not previously been diagnosed.

# 18 Cardiovascular Hazards

Cardiovascular hazards may occur during any procedure; they can be classified broadly into variations in systolic blood pressure, and cardiac arrhythmias.

## 18.1 Variations in Systolic Blood Pressure

Attitudes of anaesthetists and surgeons to changes in systolic blood pressure abound in inconsistencies. Hypotension after sympathetic blockade, either with drugs or following an epidural or subdural technique, is tolerated with equanimity, whilst falls after premedication or the induction of anaesthesia cause concern and are considered dangerous, although it is well known that systolic blood pressure falls during sleep and hence there is no reason why it should not fall after induction of anaesthesia.

### 18.1.1 Law of Poiseuille

Conventional textbooks of physiology base their teaching about pressure and flow in blood vessels on the law of Poiseuille which states that flow of Newtonian fluids through rigid tubes depends on the head of pressure and varies directly as the fourth power of the radius. If this were true for blood vessels, a graph showing the relationship between pressure and flow in blood vessels should be a straight line. Blood is not a Newtonian fluid nor are arteries rigid and in practice a pressure-flow graph for human blood vessels is not a straight line, but curved concavely, zero flow occurring before zero pressure.

The pressure at which flow stops is known as the critical closing pressure.

### 18.1.2  Law of Laplace

The law of physics relating to the flow of non-Newtonian fluids through elastic tubes is the law of Laplace, which states that the radius of a distensible tube at any given time is the result of two opposing forces: the intramural pressure distending the wall, and the tension in the wall trying to close it. This relationship can be stated as an equation in which $P$ (pressure) varies as tension over radius: $P = T/R$. At constant pressure the radius of a blood vessel and hence the quantity of fluid it can accommodate depend on variations in tension. Increase of tension reduces flow and can stop it (critical closing pressure), whilst lowering tension allows vessels to open up and increases flow.

Tension in the wall of human blood vessels is of two kinds: passive, provided by elastic tissue, which provides tension without consumption of oxygen, and active, from smooth muscle which is under nervous and hormonal control. Passive tension provided by elastic tissue permits considerable stability between transmural pressure and tension, allowing radius to vary. In order that the equation $P = T/R$ should remain stable, casual increase in pressure $P$ requires sufficient increase in tension $T$ not only to balance the increased pressure but also to contain the simultaneous expansion of the radius. Elastic tissue is able to generate more tension than is needed to meet the simultaneous demands of increased pressure and radius, and thus can maintain equilibrium of the equation $P = T/R$ without any change in radius or flow.

It is otherwise with active tension. Smooth muscle, unlike elastic tissue, is incapable of automatic stretch and thus unable to balance tension and pressure at the same time, so that tubes composed of smooth muscle are either fully open or fully shut, and no intermediate radius is possible. The reason is that a casual rise in pressure $P$ tends to increase the radius, and although tension increases to balance the pressure, it is not able to prevent the simultaneous expansion of radius. Less pressure being required to balance the tension, further increase in radius takes place, which would continue to the point of a 'blow-out', but this is prevented in practice by the fibrous tissue jacket. Conversely a casual increase in tension has the opposite effect. It overcomes pressure $P$ and decreases radius $R$. Since the decrease in radius requires less tension to balance the pressure, further decrease in radius continues until complete closure occurs. This process is somewhat difficult to understand and is sometimes called the 'bang bang' phenomenon. That is to say, tubes composed entirely of smooth muscle are either 'bang open' or 'bang shut'.

The behaviour of smooth muscle sphincters provides a verification and illustration of this theory. Sphincters contain no elastic tissue and are always either fully open or fully shut. The internal rectal sphincter is an example. It relaxes automatically when pressure increases, with incontinence if the voluntary control of the external sphincter is lost, as in paralytic lesions.

Arteriovenous shunts in the microcirculation behave in a similar fashion. Composed solely of contractile muscle cells and containing no elastic fibres, they have been shown to be either wide open or completely closed.

If the walls of small blood vessels were composed entirely of smooth muscle, regulation of blood flow would be impossible, because when vasomotor tone was high, or in the presence of circulatory catecholamines, blood vessels would behave like sphincters and close completely. However, examination of the conditions arising from a combination of active tension and passive tension shows that small blood vessels do possess a limited capacity for graded constriction, which is maximum when active tension is low and decreases as tension increases.

The Laplacian law applies particularly to the resistance vessels, the arterioles, whose walls contain a preponderance of smooth muscle and can develop considerable tension, with consequent reduction of radius. When the constriction reaches the point where the elastic fibres become slack or unstretched, passive tension no longer operates and the unstable state already described for active tension arises, and the vessels close. The pressure prevailing at the moment is known as the critical closing pressure.

Elastic tissue decreases in quantity and effectiveness with age, so that small blood vessels of elderly persons become less elastic and their capacity for graded constriction much limited. In such subjects vasoconstriction from increase in active tension (or vasomotor tone) has serious consequences. Critical closing pressure is high, and the smaller blood vessels deprived of elastic fibres tend to behave like sphincters and close at relatively high pressures. This is one reason why intense vasoconstriction in elderly subjects has such catastrophic consequences.

### 18.1.3  Law of Laplace in Clinical Practice

Application of these principles to changes in blood pressure during anaesthesia and recovery is essential if one is to appreciate their true significance. Judgement should never be passed on a fall in blood pressure without reference to perfusion and the general condition of the patient.

When low blood pressure is the result of a reduction in vasomotor tone, extremities remain warm, finger nails remain pink and the pulse is easily palpable and not rapid. Vasomotor tone and critical closing pressure are low and patients with blood pressure of about 10 kPa are in no danger.

On the other hand if a low blood pressure is accompanied by vasoconstriction with cold extremities, cyanosed nail beds, cold nose and rapid feeble pulse, the patient is in danger because venous return is impeded and cardiac output and perfusion of vital organs are inadequate. Vasomotor tone and critical closing pressure are high and with blood pressures of about 10 kPa perfusion of vital organs may become quite inadequate. In short, the condition is that usually described as 'shock'.

Hypotension from sympathetic blockade following spinal or epidural analgesia causes no harm, because critical closing pressure or vasomotor tone is low and perfusion remains adequate, as is shown by warm pink extremities. The only active treatment required is a modest intravenous infusion to compensate for the increased capacitance of the vasomotor tree. Alternatively, a slight head-down tilt will also raise systolic pressure by increasing venous return and resolve any anxieties about cerebral circulation.

Indeed, intravenous infusions were never given after spinal analgesia in the days before the introduction of disposable plastic giving sets and intravenous cannulae. The author can vouch from a wide practical experience that no harm ever resulted.

Hypotension from *central* reduction in vasomotor tone may follow premedication or induction of anaesthesia, particularly with barbiturates and halothane. Estimation of critical closing pressure in anaesthetised subjects has demonstrated the existence of a linear relationship with systolic blood pressure. This arrangement ensures consistent perfusion in spite of blood pressure changes. The simultaneous lowering of critical closing pressure with centrally induced falls in systolic pressure provides a built-in safety mechanism without which general anaesthesia would indeed be a perilous undertaking.

Hypotension from reduced vasomotor tone induced by general anaesthesia is often dramatically reversed by surgical stimulus and the sympathetic response to which it gives rise.

### 18.1.4 Operative Positions

Other causes of a fall in blood pressure are positions for operation which interfere with venous return, such as foot-down tilt and the lateral and prone positions. Kidney and gall bladder bridges can cause serious falls in pressure by interfering with venous return. When these devices are used anaesthetists should keep a careful watch after positioning of the patient and undertake frequent blood pressure estimations for the next 5-10 min.

### 18.1.5 Sudden Blood Loss

Blood loss during anaesthesia, if sudden, can result in a sudden drop in blood pressure. A less rapid fall follows progressive loss of blood, unless the loss is carefully measured and accurately replaced. Swab weighing and measurement of blood in suction bottles should be a routine procedure for all but the most minor procedures. When calculating blood loss, one must always make allowance for the blood on sterile towels and operating gowns, which can amount to as much as 30%-40% of the measured loss in major procedures such as abdominoperineal resection or radical amputation of the breast.

### 18.1.6 Shock

Haemorrhagic shock and its treatment are considered fully in Chap. 26. Bacteraemic shock can also cause fall in blood pressure during surgery. Intensive vascular spasm interferes with venous return, raises critical closing pressure and reduces perfusion. It has been observed after vigorous instrumentation of urethral strictures. Presumably breakdown of the scar tissue releases endotoxin from dead organisms and causes shock. Treatment is discussed fully in Chap. 26.

### 18.1.7 Rises in Blood Pressure

Blood pressure rises, as already noted, as part of a sympathetic response to surgical incision, the rise being more notable if a fall has taken place during induction. Rises above normal pre-operative levels may occur during exploration of the abdomen, following traction on mesenteries, or from handling the adrenal gland during mobilisation of a kidney.

Such rises are usually transient and return to normal when surgical manoeuvres cease. If they are persistent and accompanied by sweating and pallor, the vasodilation accompanying deepening of anaesthesia will lower pressure and return the patient to a more acceptable clinical state.

Blood pressure also rises in malignant hyperpyrexia, discussed in the next section.

### 18.1.8 Malignant Hyperpyrexia

Malignant hyperpyrexia is a rare condition, the outstanding features of which are muscular rigidity and a very high temperature, which can rise as quickly as 1°C every 10-15 min. The cause is unknown. Evidence exists to suggest a hereditary defect in muscle metabolism (an inability to store calcium in sarcoplasmic reticulum) and the condition is associated in several recorded instances with a raised level of serum creatinine phosphokinase—a not uncommon finding in many muscular dystrophies.

Another suggestion is that in susceptible patients the ability to convert adenosine diphosphate to triphosphate, and thus store energy for muscular contraction, is interfered with by certain anaesthetics, leading to immediate dissipation of energy in the form of heat.

*Clinical Features.* Most sufferers are young and healthy, and often the operation is minor in nature. The use of suxamethonium for intubation is a fairly constant feature, and sometimes it appears to be ineffective, leaving the jaw muscles rigid; this is said to be a helpful warning sign. Often anaesthesia proceeds normally for 30-45 min, after which pulse rate, respiratory rate and blood pressure all increase and the skin becomes hot, dry and flushed. Later this turns to cyanosis as the demand for oxygen to meet the increased metabolism outstrips the supply. These changes are accompanied by an increase in serum potassium and blood carbon dioxide and a metabolic acidosis. Unless treated energetically, death will occur from heart failure, preceded by convulsions due to cerebral damage.

*Treatment.* The operation should be suspended or brought to a speedy conclusion whilst organisation for energetic symptomatic treatment is undertaken. This should be:

1) Ventilation with 100% oxygen, with a carbon dioxide absorber in circuit

2) Infusion of sodium bicarbonate to offset metabolic acidosis

3) Cooling with ice packs, fans etc. Care should be taken, however, not to cause constriction of the veins, because this will make heat loss more difficult.

4) Procaine 0.6% intravenously. A loading dose of 30-40 mg can be given, followed by a drip of 0.2 mg/kg/min, to reduce muscle rigidity and drive calcium back into the cells.

This last raises the question whether a central nervous disturbance could be involved, since procaine is a known depressant of the medullary brain stem reticular formation, the site of the facilitatory centre controlling muscle tone. If this is so, then the use of chlorpromazine in this condition could be seriously considered. It dilates veins, increases heat loss and relaxes muscles by a depressant action on the facilitatory centre in the medullary reticular formation.

Recent reports claim that a skeletal muscle relaxant, dantrolene (Dantrium), is superior to procaine in prevention (when a raised creatinine phosphokinase level indicates risk) and in treatment. The drug is said to act by interfering with release of calcium from sarcoplasm and directly inhibits development of contractile tension at a point distal to the myoneural junction. The preparation is expensive and becomes ineffective after storage for two years. Side-effects related to dose and duration of treatment include hepatitis, muscular weakness, constipation and bowel obstruction, slurred speech, ataxia, blurred vision, nausea and vomiting. The list is formidable, but it is comforting to know that they are said to be minimal if the recommended dosage (0.8 mg/kg) is not exceeded.

*Prevention.* Suggestions that suxamethonium and halothane trigger off the condition have not been substantiated. The condition does not appear for 30-45 min, by which time metabolism of suxamethonium is complete. That suxamethonium and halothane should occur so frequently in reported cases is not surprising as they are the most commonly used agents in anaesthesia. Where a hereditary factor is suspected, blood relatives should be warned, and a screen for resting levels of serum creatinine phosphokinase should be made.

## 18.2  Cardiac Arrhythmias

Cardiac irregularities are not uncommon during anaesthesia, as the increasing routine use of cardioscopes has revealed. The commonest irregularity is an extrasystole, usually associated with increase in activity of the sympathetic nervous system. An extrasystole can appear in apprehensive patients even before anaesthesia begins, and apprehension itself predisposes to cardiac irregularity. Once anaesthesia has been induced, the commonest causes are accumulation of carbon dioxide in the bloodstream from respiratory depression, and increased sympathetic activity from surgical stimulation, particularly in sensitive areas such as the ocular muscles, the tympanic membrane and the upper abdomen. The use of adrenaline or cocaine by surgeons for vasoconstriction is another cause. It is said by surgeons that subcutaneous injection of adrenaline in saline at a strength of 1:100 000 or 10% cocaine placed in the nose will not cause disturbance, but many anaesthetists doubt this.

Anaesthetic agents also make a contribution to cardiac arrhythmias. Ether and cyclopropane, for example, are stimulants of sympathetic activity, though irregularities are rare with ether. Halothane, too, has been implicated, although the evidence is contradictory, as it is said to antagonise sympathetic activity in the heart, and one would not expect in these circumstances to encounter arrhythmias. Halothane does cause a slowing of the pulse (bradycardia) which should always be reversed by intravenous injection of 0.6 mg atropine if the rate falls to 50 or below. Bradycardia has far more potential danger than tachycardia.

Endotracheal intubation after administration of suxamethonium produces arrhythmias reflexly in 60% of patients owing to disturbance of vagal nerve endings. Sympathetic antagonists such as droperidol and chlorpromazine when used as premedication reduce the incidence.

*Oculocardiac Reflex.* Stimuli in or near the eye or traction on ocular muscles (especially the internal rectus) result in cardiac irregularity in the form of extrasystoles and bradycardia. Cardiac arrest may result. Preventative measures include routine inclusion of atropine in premedication and ensuring that adequate depth of anaesthesia is reached. Before surgery begins, the patient should be in the first plane of third stage of anaesthesia (Guedel), i.e. with the eyes symmetrical and central.

Other abnormal rhythms occurring during anaesthesia include:

*Sinus arrhythmia* (pulse slowing on expiration), commoner in the conscious stage and related to increased vagal tone, usually disappears as anaesthesia deepens.

*Pulsus paradoxus* (the converse of sinus arrhythmia, with slowing on inspiration) can be the result of too powerful mechanical ventilation interfering with venous return.

*Pulsus alternans* occurs when one strong beat is followed by a weak one, and poses problems in blood pressure readings since at higher pressures only the stronger stimulus appears, giving the impression of bradycardia. A change to tachycardia occurs when the weaker beat appears, at a lower pressure. The phenomenon is associated with high pulse rates (paroxysmal tachycardia) and auricular flutter.

*Pulsus bigeminus* or 'coupling' of beats arises from an extrasystole immediately following a normal beat, after which the heart muscle remains refractory, so that there is an interval before the next beat. Two normal beats followed by an extrasystole not picked up at the wrist produce the same effects.

*Treatment* of arrhythmias should be conservative initially. Surgeons should be asked to stop stimulation to allow hyperventilation (to lower excess carbon dioxide) and deepening anaesthesia to take effect.

If simple measures fail, intravenous injection of 1-2 mg propranolol (a beta-blocker) will slow the heart and restore normal rhythm. A 1% solution of lignocaine given intravenously in a dose of 1 mg/kg body weight is also effective. It is said to reduce arrhythmia by direct action on heart muscle, but there is considerable evidence that it may also do so by a central action.

# 19 Controlled Hypotension

Although smooth anaesthesia and avoidance of venous congestion by posture help to reduce bleeding, there are occasions when anaesthetists deliberately produce hypotension. This technique, known as induced or controlled hypotension, is undertaken to facilitate delicate surgery of the middle ear and removal of highly vascular tumours, as well as for certain plastic, gynaecological, urological and orthopaedic operations. Methods which have been used include differential spinal anaesthesia and arteriotomy, but these will not be discussed in this chapter, which only deals with the use of the ganglion blocking agents, i.e. hexamethonium (Vegolysen), pentolinium (Ansolysen) and trimetaphan (Arfonad), which relax smooth muscle coats of blood vessels, and sodium nitroprusside which paralyses them.

There are several hazards of controlled hypotension, but the greatest are lack of experience by the anaesthetist and poor communication with the surgeon. Hazards arise (a) from the agents (particularly sodium nitroprusside), (b) from reduced perfusion of vital organs (especially the central nervous system), (c) from reactionary haemorrhage, (d) from wrong choice of patient and (e) from use in the wrong type of operation.

### 19.1  Factors Involved in Reducing Bleeding

Reduced bleeding results partly from lowered blood pressure and partly from unimpeded drainage of blood from the operation site into widely dilated veins, which is assisted by posture; also, since up to 75% of blood volume can be accommodated in dilated veins, fall in cardiac output also contributes to reduction of systolic pressure.

Posture should be so arranged as to ensure free and unimpeded venous drainage of the operation site and can be head-down or foot-down, according to the circumstances.

Venous congestion must be kept to a minimum and coughing avoided, ideally by controlled respiration, which however removes a vital sign of respiratory failure from medullary anaemia due to excessive fall in blood pressure and should be avoided by the inexperienced, especially with a patient in a foot-down position.

### 19.2  Ganglion Blocking Agents

Hexamethonium (10-40 mg) and pentolinium (5-10 mg) are given intravenously after induction of anaesthesia, but trimetaphan, whose action is of short duration, requires a continuous intravenous infusion of 1 mg/ml at about 60 drops per minute. The total dose at any time should never exceed 1 g (or 1 litre of fluid).

Ganglionic blockade affects both sympathetic and parasympathetic ganglia, and so additional effects include dilatation of the pupils, retention of urine and tachycardia.

### 19.3  Sodium Nitroprusside

The drug is prepared in 0.01% solution. The dose varies between 2.5 and 100 mg/h, but the total dose should never exceed 200 mg.

#### 19.3.1  Resistance

In many units, if satisfactory low blood pressure does not follow infusion of 50 mg over 30 min, the method is abandoned, because patients (especially young adults) are resistant. Resistance to the hypotensive effect of ganglion blocking agents and sodium nitroprusside occurs principally in young subjects. A possible explanation is the relatively rich supply of elastic tissue in the arterioles of younger age groups, which provides considerable residual tension or peripheral resistance, in spite of complete relaxation of smooth muscle. The temptation to push dosage should be resisted, but a slight increase in foot-down tilt to encourage venous drainage may help to reduce bleeding.

### 19.3.2   Toxic Effects

Sodium nitroprusside is broken down by liver rodanase into sodium thiocyanate, which is converted to free cyanide by the thiocyanate oxidase in red blood corpuscles. The resulting hydrocyanic acid is excreted through the lungs, detectable as an odour of bitter almonds. Blood thiocyanate above 15-20 mg/100 ml exceeds the detoxifying powers of the body, and cyanide accumulates, neutralising cytochrome oxidase, vital for oxygen utilisation by cells, so that acute anoxia results. This action is reversible, but only if recognised early.

After administration of a fatal dose, signs of overdose do not occur for at least half an hour, when respiration becomes irregular and sighing, respiratory failure, coma and cardiac arrest occur in a further half hour.

### 19.3.3   Treatment for Overdose

Following any change in respiratory pattern during recovery, a sample of blood should be taken immediately for estimation of thiocyanate level. The object of treatment is to give drugs which form methaemoglobin, which absorbs cyanide and prevents union with cytochrome oxidase. This can be brought about by inhalation of amylnitrite followed by intravenous infusion of sodium nitrite. Intravenous injection of dicobalt tetracemate (Kelocyanor), which behaves like methaemoglobin, is a simpler and better procedure. An intraveous injection of 2 ampoules followed by 50 ml hypertonic glucose (strong dextrose BPC) should restore normal blood pressure and breathing. Treatment is unpleasant but never fatal.

During treatment of cyanide poisoning, patients should receive 100% oxygen by mechanical ventilation. It has been reported that a patient who had intentionally taken a fatal dose of cyanide recovered following energetic treatment with 100% oxygen and intravenous fluids.

Sodium nitroprusside should never be used to induce hypotension by anyone unfamiliar with the method. Ideally two anaesthetists should be present and doses carefully checked. At least two fatalities from overdose have been recorded. It must be remembered that the signs of overdose may not become evident for half an hour after the end of the administration.

### 19.3.4   Other Uses

Sodium nitroprusside has also been used with benefit for acute coronary thrombosis and for treatment of intractable high blood pressure.

## 19.4   Effects of Reduced Perfusion

### 19.4.1   Heart

Fears of an adverse effect on cardiac function from hypotension have not proved justified.

Although coronary perfusion decreases, this is more than compensated for by the reduced work of the heart and reduced oxygen consumption. The law of Laplace also applies to the heart, and tension developed prior to contraction accounts for much of the oxygen requirement.

### 19.4.2 Brain

Suggestions that hypotension has adverse effects on cerebral function have not been confirmed.

Cerebral thrombosis is rare, but has occurred in association with local pre-existing arterial disease or cerebrovascular abnormality. These complications are not encountered in plastic units, in one of which no cerebral changes were reported in over 9000 patients receiving controlled hypotension.

When a foot-down tilt is used, allowance must be made for the height of the column of blood between the brain and the point where pressure is measured on the arm, for there is a reduction of about 0.1 kPa pressure for every centimetre in height difference between the arm and the head. In a fairly steep foot-down tilt this could amount to 30-40 cm (3-4 kPa) and thus convert a blood pressure of 9.5 kPa at the arm to one as low as 5.5 kPa at the brain level.

### 19.4.3 Lungs

Hypotension decreases pulmonary efficiency and is evident as an increase in alveolar dead space. The resulting increase in $P_{CO_2}$ benefits the brain, as it improves cerebral circulation. Otherwise no pulmonary complications have been reported.

### 19.4.4 Kidneys

Decrease in renal blood flow is less than expected during controlled hypotension. Urine flow is said to cease at a blood pressure of 9.3 kPa, but continues below this figure if vasodilatation is present. Any adverse renal changes (oliguria 0.19% or anuria 0.22%) have occurred chiefly in urological units when the method has been used for prostatectomy or total cystectomy. Possibly these patients had some defect of renal function before their operations.

### 19.4.5 Liver

No reports of liver damage have been made.

### 19.4.6 Retina

Thrombosis of the retinal artery is a rare complication. It has been reported where the artery was diseased (a contra-indication) and when too steep a foot-down tilt was used.

## 19.5  Reactionary Haemorrhage

The main surgical hazard to controlled hypotension is reactionary haemorrhage, particularly after surgery of the prostate, bladder or breast. The best preventative measure is to allow pressure to rise gradually towards the conclusion of the operation, so that the surgeon can deal with bleeding points which become evident.

## 19.6  Wrong Choice of Patient

Certain classes of patients are unsuitable for hypotensive technique. Presence of arteriosclerosis in any form, whether coronary, cerebrovascular or of a major artery, is a contra-indication, because it is so often a manifestation of a general atheromatous change throughout the body, and it means also that some of the main arterial channels may be blocked by rigid atheromatous plaques. These confer a rigidity which justifies the application of Poiseuille's law to flow problems. Reduced radius means serious reduction of flow at low pressure, a greater reduction than would occur in the absence of obstruction with the presence of elastic tension. Any condition which interferes with oxygen consumption, e.g. anaemia or respiratory disease, is also an obvious contra-indication.

## 19.7  Use in Wrong Type of Operation

Opinions differ about which operations should be included for controlled hypotension. This is a personal matter between anaesthetist and surgeon. Major plastic surgery and maxillofacial operations, mainly performed on young, relatively fit patients, stand very high on the list of suitability. Prostatectomy and breast surgery come low on the list, because satisfactory conditions can more easily be produced with halothane. For prostate and bladder surgery, epidural or subdural techniques ensure minimal blood loss with far less danger of reactionary haemorrhage and haematoma formation than when controlled hypotension is used. Controlled hypotension has many advocates for middle ear and neurosurgery. Much depends on the attitude of surgical colleagues. It must always be remembered, too, that induced hypotension for head and neck surgery carries greater risk of permanent neurological damage than hypotension in more dependent parts, when the head can be kept low.

# 20 Intravenous Therapy and Central Venous Pressure Lines

## 20.1. Intravenous Therapy

### 20.1.1 Examination of Solutions

Solutions of dextran and electrolytes should always be examined against a bright light before use, to exclude the presence of any foreign material or crystals. Solutions showing any abnormality should be discarded. Some may be infected, others may contain foreign material, which can cause a pyrexial reaction, and others may contain inert particles, which can cause small emboli. When solutions of electrolytes or dextran are administered, their batch numbers should be entered in the patient's record, to enable tracing the batch if any adverse reaction occurs.

### 20.1.2 Plasma Substitutes

Dextran 110, 70 and 40 are recommended for treatment of acute haemorrhage until whole blood is available if plasma solutions (e.g. plasma protein fraction) cannot be obtained. Since dextran solutions interfere with blood grouping tests, adequate samples of blood should be taken for this purpose before administration. The large molecules of dextran 110 can block renal tubules, but those of lower molecular weight (70) leave the circulation sooner. Dextran 70 is the most widely used dextran but does prolong bleeding time and should be used with caution if there are abnormalities in the patient's clotting mechanism.

### 20.1.3 Electrolyte Infusion

Three main hazards to infusion of electrolytes are sodium excess, potassium excess and water excess.

*Sodium excess* is evidenced by oedema of dependent parts and moist sounds in the lungs, often following enthusiastic electrolyte infusion during and after surgery. Retention of sodium is maximum for the first 48 h after operation owing to antidiuretic hormone secretion, which reduces urine output to less than 500 ml for 24 h.

*Potassium excess* may follow too free administration of potassium salt to patients with suspected deficiencies or, more commonly, in patients with disturbed kidney function, especially after large blood transfusions. The effect of potassium becomes evident in the electrocardiogram as a disturbance of the conductive system; early signs are a high T wave followed by reduction of the R wave. The T wave later reduces in size with deepening of the notch of the S wave. Terminally, ventricular fibrillation may occur.

Patients with oliguria or renal disease should not receive potassium. If low blood potassium is suspected, potassium by mouth, e.g. in fruit drinks, is safer than by the intravenous route. When it is necessary to give potassium intravenously, 1 g potassium chloride is added to 500 ml of 5% dextrose solution and given slowly. The maximum amount which a patient should received in 24 h is 6 g.

If there is electrocardiographic evidence of cardiac intoxication, 100 ml of 50% glucose and 10 units of insulin should be given by the intravenous route. Since a low blood sodium or calcium can intensify the toxic effects of excess potassium, the above solution should be followed by 10 ml of 10% calcium gluconate and 250 ml of 1.4% sodium bicarbonate.

*Water intoxication* may follow injudicious infusion of 10% glucose dissolved in water, by either the intravenous or the rectal route, to a patient who is already taking fluids by mouth. Since the excess water is distributed equally between the extracellular, intracellular and circulatory compartments, physical signs such as congested neck veins and moist lung sounds are absent. The main effect of excess water in the brain is swelling of the brain cells, evident as lethargy, headache and disorientation, accompanied by cramps in the muscles (probably central in the origin) and, later, convulsions. Examination of the electrolyte content of the tissue fluids will reveal that the sodium level is very low, and other evidence of haemodilution may be present. The condition is quickly reversible by administration of hypertonic saline, for example 500 ml of 5% sodium chloride.

## 20.1.4 Additives to Intravenous Fluids

In some hospitals as many as one patient in three receives some additive to an intravenous infusion and one in six receives more than one drug. One in every six patients receives drugs which are incompatible either with the infusion fluid or with each other. Responsibility is left to nursing staff, who are seldom provided with clear instructions or the means of recording what they inject.

Owing to the risk of degradation, drugs should not be added to infusions of:

1) Blood, plasma or other blood products
2) Parenteral amino acids or lipid preparations
3) Infusions of mannitol or sodium bicarbonate

When adding to infusions of other fluids, drugs should be checked (if necessary with a pharmacist) for compatibility.

The more common incompatibilities are set out in Table 2. Adequate mixing of solutions is essential, especially when specific gravities vary. Multiple drug additions should be avoided whenever possible. The risk of deleterious physical or chemical changes increases: the therapeutic response may be altered, both agents may be inactivated, and harmful by-products may be produced.

**Table 2.** Incompatibilities of drugs added to intravenous infusions

| | |
|---|---|
| Do not add drugs to the following: | Amino acid solutions<br>Lipid mixtures<br>Mannitol solutions—check solution has not yet crystallised<br>Blood and blood products |
| Potassium chloride | Normally not more than 80 mmol $K^+$ (6 g potassium chloride) should be infused in 24 h |
| Penicillins | Add only to sodium chloride 0.9% solution and prepare immediately before administration |
| Ampicillin | No other drug to be added to infusion |
| Cephaloridine | Tetracyclines, erythromycin incompatible |
| Chloramphenicol | Tetracyclines, hydrocortisone incompatible |
| Erythromycin lactobionate | Add only to dextrose 5%, not electrolyte solutions<br>No other drugs to be added to infusion |
| Heparin | Add preferably to sodium chloride 0.9% solution<br>Antibiotics, hydrocortisone, incompatible |
| Hydrocortisone sodium succinate | Antibiotics, heparin incompatible |
| Iron dextran | See manufacturer's literature |
| Tetracyclines | No other drugs to be added to infusion<br>Do not add to solution containing calcium |
| Compound vitamin injection | Inadvisable to add a multiple constituent injection to an infusion |

Consult the pharmacy department about other drugs to be added to an infusion solution. Remember to affix a 'drug additive' label to each infusion with an additive.

Every hospital should have procedures for administration of intravenous fluids agreed by doctors, nurses and pharmacists. There should be regular educational sessions for new members of nursing and medical staff on agreed procedures and ways of avoiding hazards.

The commonest additions to intavenous fluid are:

1) Potassium chloride, for electrolyte disturbances
2) Heparin, to prevent blood clotting and to treat thrombosis
3) Lignocaine, for treatment of cardiac arrhythmias
4) Antiobiotics, for treatment of acute infection
5) Corticosteroids, for shock, arthritis, asthma, Crohn's disease, etc.
6) Vitamins, for malnutrition
7) Oxytocin, in midwifery, for induction of childbirth

The intravenous route should only be used when there is a very clear indication and when the intramuscular and oral routes are impossible. When it is decided to administer a drug intravenously, clear written instructions are necessary to ensure the desired concentration is reached and maintained. Additions may be continuous or intermittent.

*Continuous* infusion is only indicated if the drug is well diluted in order to maintain a constant therapeutic action, e.g. potassium chloride, heparin, lignocaine or oxytocin. Potassium chloride is added to infusion fluid during manufacture, in solution containing 20 or 40 mmol potassium/litre. Heparin made up in a small volume is best given from a disposable syringe by means of a motorised pump. Lignocaine is added to dextrose or fructose solutions during manufacture. Continuous oxytocin drips are administered to speed up childbirth.

*Intermittent* injection is the best way to give antibiotics, since the intravenous route presents difficulties in maintaining a steady concentration. Intramuscular and oral routes are preferable and achieve more constant blood levels. Vitamins can be given by intermittent injection but they are hardly ever necessary. Steroids are better given by the intramuscular route, although the intravenous route is used for the large dose for treatment of bacterial shock.

There are several ways of giving intermittent intravenous injections, each of which has its own drawback:

1) Puncture of the rubber bulb at the injection site is commonly used. Although convenient, leakage and infection may occur after multiple injections.

2) Incorporation of a burette into the intravenous set reduces the chance of infection but has practical difficulties.

3) Injection through a scalp vein needle or cannula also carries some risk of infection and blood may clot in the needle between injections.

4) Injection through the side arm of a three-way tap is a good method and reduces infection to a minimum.

5) When a large volume has to be infused, a second infusion set is linked to the main line by a Y-piece or a needle; a common and useful method.

Table 2 lists some of the more commonly used intravenous additives, with recommendations about their administration.

*Documentation.* Poor documentation is a hazard for patients and nursing staff. Documents for recording intravenous fluids should be available in all hospitals. Written instructions should be legible, clear and unambiguous. A record of every drug added must be maintained and filed with the patient's notes, not destroyed when the patient is discharged.

*Identification of Additives.* Each infusion container must carry a label clearly indicating the name of the patient, the name and dose of the drug and the date and time when added.

*Responsibilities of Doctors.* Medical staff are responsible for ordering additives and must

1) Ensure the additive is suitable for administration and compatible with the fluid, consulting a pharmacist when in doubt

2) Decide how it should be added

3) Write instructions clearly, including the name of the drug, the dose, and the method and rate of administration.

*Responsibilities of Nurses.* Opinions differ about how far a nurse should be held responsible for intravenous additives. There is general agreement that registered or qualified nurses who have received appropriate training in the procedure may add medicaments to intravenous infusions. The same applies to state certified midwives. These fluids may be administered by nurses in training under the supervision of a qualified trained nurse, but they should never be given by nursing auxiliaries. The responsibility of nurses also includes (a) checking the container for faults and contamination, (b) checking that the correct patient receives the fluid prescribed, (c) general supervision of the infusion, especially for patency of the cannula and rate of flow, (d) reporting immediately any abnormal response or any unexpected change in the patient's condition.

## 20.2 Central Venous Pressure Lines

Measurement of central venous pressure (CVP) is undertaken frequently during anaesthesia for cardiac and major vascular surgery, in intensive care units to control replacement of fluids after severe haemorrhage, to assess effectiveness of fluid replacement in shock states and hypovolaemia due to fluid loss, and also in treatment of left ventricular failure. Recently it has become a popular route for intravenous feeding of cachectic patients.

Central venous pressure lines may be inserted either through the median basilic vein in the elbow, or suprasternally through the internal jugular vein, or just below the clavicle through the subclavian vein. The technical details of insertion are included in all standard textbooks of anaesthesia published after 1972; readers should consult them before attempting this manoeuvre. The hazards of these procedures are by no means negligible and should encourage a conservative attitude in their use.

Hazards are of two kinds, those related to the actual insertion and those arising from the presence of an indwelling venous catheter in a blood vessel in the chest and close to the heart.

Hazards during insertion include: pneumothorax (especially following subclavian approach), hydromediastinum, subcutaneous emphysema, injury to brachial plexus (suprasternal approach), laceration of veins, subclavian artery puncture and haematoma. In addition to this imposing catalogue, hazards of a catheter in situ include infection, air embolus, hydrothorax, and cardiac tamponade following perforation of pericardium, right atrium or right ventricle. The three most serious hazards are cardiac tamponade, hydromediastinum and infection.

### 20.2.1  Cardiac Tamponade

The greatest immediate danger is that of cardiac tamponade. Rapid diagnosis is the only way of avoiding cardiac arrest. It should be suspected in any patient with a CVP line who *suddenly* complains of nausea or epigastric discomfort or who becomes confused with dyspnoea, tachycardia, fall in blood pressure and sudden increase in CVP with distended neck veins. Failure of the CVP line to fluctuate with respiration is a suspicious clinical sign. If it is accompanied by failure to aspirate blood through the catheter and a sudden rise in CVP, a diagnosis of cardiac tamponade is justified. Diagnosis may be confirmed by results of aspiration through the catheter. Failure to aspirate anything means that the catheter is certainly outside the vein; aspiration of clear or blood-stained fluid should bring immediate relief, and when no more fluid can be obtained, the catheter should be withdrawn.

If clinical deterioration continues, direct pericardial aspiration should be performed without delay. A needle suitable for this purpose should be included in every pack set up for insertion of CVP lines or kept ready sterilised wherever CVP lines are inserted. Should pericardial aspiration fail to relieve the patient, then a diagnosis of hydromediastinum should be considered.

### 20.2.2  Hydromediastinum

*Hydromediastinum* can occur when the CVP line perforates the vein. The symptoms are increasing difficulty in breathing and cyanosis during or immediately after infusion of 0.5-1.0 litre of fluid. A portable X-ray apparatus or, better still, an image-intensifier is essential for making a quick differential diagnosis in patients in respiratory distress. Aspiration of the injected fluid is both a diagnostic and a therapeutic measure and should bring relief. If the symptoms continue after withdrawal of fluid, an X-ray of the chest will show whether there is residual fluid or pneumothorax.

### 20.2.3  Infection

Infection varies between mild sepsis at the insertion site and extensive cellulitis of the neck, involving cranial nerves. Placement of the catheter requires sterile equipment and full aseptic technique. Daily dressing of the puncture site with standard antiseptics (iodine or chlorhexidine) is an efficient prophylactic measure. Withdrawal of the catheter within 48 h is certain to prevent infection.

When patients have positive blood cultures, the organisms may colonize on the catheter tip; cultures obtained in this way do not necessarily indicate failure of aseptic technique.

### 20.2.4  Prevention of Complications

As in so many other procedures, inexperience is a main reason for immediate complications (pneumothorax, haematoma formation, brachial plexus injury, etc.) as well as for later complications such as cardiac tamponade. Inexperienced junior staff are entitled to expect supervision and help from a senior colleague for their first few attempts. If a single-handed attempt is unavoidable, approach via the left median basilic vein is the simplest and surest method, provided X-ray control is available.

*Correct Placement.*  The need for accurate placement cannot be over-stated. In one series of 300 patients, the catheter tip was located in the right atrium or right ventricle in 13% of patients. The catheter tip should come to rest not more than 2 cm below a line joining the lower surfaces of the inner ends of the two clavicles. Radiographic confirmation is essential, either by use of a radio-opaque catheter or injection of 2 ml of a contrast medium such as Conray 60. Patients with catheters in an arm vein should be X-rayed with the arm abducted to a right angle and told *not* to raise the arm above that level under any circumstances, as this would push the catheter end into the right atrium.

Once in position, the end of the catheter at the puncture site must be secured firmly with tape and adhesive plaster to reduce movement to a minimum. Perforation of the superior vena cava, right atrium or ventricle by the catheter tip is more likely if a rigid bevel tip comes into contact with the pulsatile walls of the heart. Even soft tips, however, can pass through these structures, and even when the tip is correctly placed, movement can occur as the result of blood flow, pressure changes transmitted from the heart, and the action of muscles and joints through or over. which the catheter passes. For this reason no injection should be made into a CVP line without previous aspiration of blood.

*Type of Catheter.* Preferably catheters should be radio-opaque, soft and pliable, and should not remain in place for more than 48 h. All reported cases of cardiac tamponade and infection have occurred after this period.

# 21 Blood Transfusion

Opinions differ about the incidence and severity of complications following blood transfusion. Some authorities place mortality as high as 1 in 1000 and the incidence of undesirable reactions at 5%. Other authorities claim mortality is negligible and entirely avoidable by observing basic rules, whilst admitting that minor reactions are unavoidable but of little significance compared with the value of transfusing patients. Careful preparation, cross-matching and storage have reduced reactions in countries with well-organised, adequately equipped and properly supervised blood transfusion services.

The following complications may occur during transfusion:

1) Febrile reaction

2) Circulatory overload

3) Haemolysis (usually from infusion of incompatible blood)

4) Air embolism

5) Infection

6) Cardiac arrest

7) Allergic responses

8) Complications due to faulty addition of medicaments

## 21.1 Febrile Reaction

Three types of febrile reaction are described:

Grade I, mild—rise of temperature to 37.8°C

Grade II, moderate—rise of temperature above 37.8°C, with a sense of chill

Grade III, severe—sudden rise of temperature to about 40°C, accompanied by rigors

The usual cause of reaction is the presence of pyrogens in the blood; this should be distinguished from fluctuation in patients' temperature in the course of the illness. Another, rarer cause of pyrexia is presence of white cell antibodies; those affected should receive 'leucocyte-poor' blood.

During Grade I and II reactions infusions should continue, but an antipyretic (aspirin) or, better, an antihistamine should be prescribed.

Grade III reaction with rigors is an indication for stopping the infusion.

## 21.2 Circulatory Overload

Overload of the circulation becomes obvious when the neck veins become congested, accompanied by difficulty in breathing, indicating oedema of the lungs. Too rapid infusion in normovolaemic subjects can precipitate the condition. Patients with heart disease and compensated anaemia are particularly prone and should only be given packed cells slowly, the rate of infusion never exceeding 40 drops per minute. Infusion should stop if signs of overload appear, and excess fluid should be reduced with diuretics.

## 21.3 Haemolysis

A haemolytic reaction can occur from transfusion of incompatible blood, from outdated blood or from blood which has been haemolysed by freezing, overheating or bacterial contamination.

### 21.3.1 Incompatibility

The commonest cause of incompatibility is failure to check that the blood used is that intended for that patient. It is standard practice to make sure the name and hospital number on the blood pack is the same as on the identity band of the patient, whilst the number on the blood unit must agree with the number indicated on the grouping sheet from the blood tranfusion laboratory.

Every year fatal accidents occur from failure to observe these simple precautions. One source of confusion arises when a patient receives in the ward an emergency transfusion cross-matched for another patient of the *same name.* Hence the need to check number as well as name. Incompatible transfusion can follow indiscriminate use of group O (universal blood). Some group O donors have sufficient antibodies to destroy cells of either AB or A or B recipients and produce a haemolytic reaction. The use of O Rhesus-negative blood for a Rhesus-positive patient who may have been immunised to one of the Rhesus subgroups can occasionally cause haemolysis. Despite these drawbacks, where a delay would endanger life, the use of O Rhesus-negative blood certified free from dangerous A or B antibodies is permissible.

### 21.3.2  Stored Blood

A normal container of blood shows a clear line of demarcation between cells and the plasma, which is straw-coloured. Suspicion of haemolysis in blood should arise if examination of a container shows reddish discoloration of plasma above the cell layer gradually spreading upwards. Plasma bags should be stored upright in order to observe the condition of the plasma. Haemolysis may be present in outdated blood (more than 14 days old). The expiratory date is marked on each container.

Variations in temperature—either extreme heat or extreme cold—induce haemolysis, for which reason domestic refrigerators are not suitable for the storage of blood, which must be stored in a specially designed refrigerator (British Standard 4376/1968) which maintains blood at a temperature between 4°C and 6°C. A medically qualified person should be held responsible for its maintenance. The internal temperature is recorded on the outside and an alarm operates if temperature exceeds 6°C or becomes less than 4°C.

### 21.3.3  Diagnosis

A febrile reaction during transfusion should always be considered a warning of possible haemolysis and a reason to discontinue the infusion. Breathlessness, headache, sensation of constriction in the chest, or pain in the back are more definite signs that haemolysis is taking place. None of these appear during anaesthesia, which explains why transfusion is withheld in some centres until consciousness returns.

Later signs appearing with recovery of consciousness are (in increasing order of severity):

1) Haemoglobinuria

2) Oligaemic shock, i.e. vasoconstriction, low blood pressure, sweating and pallor

3) Incipient renal failure, as shown by reduction or cessation of urine output and increase in the serum sodium, urea and creatinine

4) Soon after (3), multiple haemorrhage arising from acute defibrination syndrome

5) Jaundice, which may be delayed for as long as 48 h

### 21.3.4 Treatment

The aim of treatment should be threefold:

1) To reduce the injury or stress response caused by action of the degraded red cells on the central nervous system

2) To treat the oligaemic shock which is a consequence of the above

3) To improve the function of the kidney whose output is reduced by (a) vasoconstriction of the glomeruli, or (b) blocking of the tubules by haemoglobin, which escapes through the ruptured capillaries of the glomeruli.

The intensity of the stress response and consequent oligaemic shock can be reduced or reversed by intravenous chlorpromazine diluted in saline and given slowly up to an amount of 50 mg, or by a bolus injection of 1 g hydrocortisone. Infusion of Hartmann's solution to reduce blood viscosity and improve perfusion of the kidney is preferable to blood, plasma or plasma protein fractions. The above measures will contribute to restoration of renal secretion.

In addition to its vasodilator action, chlorpromazine also antagonises release of the antidiuretic hormone and helps to increase urine output.

During treatment, a fluid balance chart is essential, and in the absence of a satisfactory renal output, restriction of intravenous fluids is advisable, especially when venous pressure rises, as seen by engorgement of the neck veins or through a central venous pressure line. If kidney function does not improve, acute renal failure is probable and may be confirmed by the following measures: a plasma potassium figure of more than 6 mmol/l, signs of hyperkalaemia in the electrocardiogram and urine sodium greater than 20 mmol/l, and increased blood urea. Most severe haemolytic reactions go into renal failure, which should be assumed when the urine output is less than 400-500 ml in 24 h. In such circumstances, prophylactic dialysis may prevent the onset of uraemia and will allow adequate intake of protein and calories by the patient.

## 21.4  Air Embolism

### 21.4.1  Causes

During rapid transfusion after massive haemorrhage (during a surgical operation or following major injury), some means of increasing the infusion pressure becomes necessary. It should never be done by forcing air directly into the vessel containing blood, because when it becomes empty (as it does very rapidly) air enters the infusion tubing and the venous circulation, with serious risk of air embolism. Modern infusion sets contain a ball in the drip chamber which obstructs exit of air when the container becomes empty, and thus provides a built-in insurance against air embolism. There are two other, safer ways of speeding perfusion flow. First, manual compression or enclosure in a pressure bag will ensure rapid emptying of plastic containers. On no account should an air vent be put into plastic containers, because introducing air renders air embolus possible. Second, rapid infusion from solid containers is obtained by a rotary pump fitted onto the infusion tubing distal to the drip chamber.

Other sources of air embolus are leaks in infusion tubing, and direct infusion of a second intravenous fluid into the rubber connection at the end of the giving set if the container has an air vent.

### 21.4.2  Signs and Symptoms

It is not until a considerable quantity of air has entered the circulation that signs and symptoms manifest themselves. If detected early, the leak can be sealed before the appearance of significant signs, which are: deepening of respiration and coughing, followed by unconsciousness and cardiovascular failure. A classical, but late, sign is 'water-wheel murmur' over the heart, which has been descibed as a 'churning and splashing' sound.

### 21.4.3  Treatment

A head-down position will encourage bubbles of air in the veins to pass upwards to the pelvic and leg veins where they are harmless. Placing the patient on the *left* side will allow air in the right ventricle to pass towards the apex, thus preventing formation of an air lock at the pulmonary aortic valve.

Artificial respiration should be performed with 100% oxygen. A wide-bore needle is passed into the distended jugular vein for withdrawal of any blood-stained froth present. A similar puncture and aspiration of froth of the right ventricle should be performed.

As a last resort, an emergency thoracotomy should be performed and aspiration of the right ventricle undertaken under direct vision.

## 21.5  Infected Blood

### 21.5.1  Bacterial Infection

Infection from stored blood is very rare. The symptoms resemble a haemolytic reaction and can only be distinguished by blood culture. It is more than likely that the reticulo-endothelial system would deal with any injected bacteria. Some authorities maintain that bacteria do not multiply in the bloodstream and that septicaemia with a positive blood culture only arises if there is some breeding-place, such as a thrombus in a vein, or vegetation on a cardiac valve.

### 21.5.2  Serum Hepatitis

Two viral agents are known to cause hepatitis. Hepatitis A virus causes infectious hepatitis and hepatitis B, also known as Australia antigen, causes serum hepatitis. As hepatitis B is found in the bloodstream it can be transmitted from infected donors and via all contaminated products from contaminated blood, with the exception of plasma protein fraction and human albumin, which are treated by heat to 60°C for 10 h, long enought to destroy the antigen.

All blood donors are screened for hepatitis B antigen and about 1:1000 found to have it. Screening has reduced the incidence of serum hepatitis by a quarter but, as tests are not completely foolproof, a small risk continues, estimated at 0.15% for each unit of blood. Apart from transmission of serum hepatitis to patients by blood transfusion, the presence of hepatitis B antigen in unsymptomatic carriers who are patients constitutes a separate hazard for their medical and nursing attendants since the virus, being present in the blood, can also be transmitted by personal contact. Certain classes of patients are said to have a higher chance of carrying the antigen. These include patients undergoing haemodialysis, patients with leukaemia, reticuloses, or liver disease, and those whose resistance has been lowered by radiotherapy, treatment with cytotoxic agents, or immunosuppressive drugs.

When hepatitis B is known or suspected to be present in a patient, all operating personnel coming into contact should wear disposable gloves, gowns and masks and use only disposable products during the operation, all of which should be destroyed at the end by fire. Anaesthetists and their assistants must take particular care to avoid contamination from shed blood when setting up intravenous infusions. The same considerations apply in those nursing staff who handle the blood-stained swabs and drapes during operation.

Clinically, serum hepatitis is indistinguishable from infective hepatitis. The incubation period of serum hepatitis can be as long as 180 days and this, no doubt in several instances, makes clinical differential diagnosis almost impossible.

### 21.5.3  Other Types of Infection

Blood from donors can also convey infections such as syphilis and parasitic diseases, especially malaria. Blood transfusion services submit donors to careful screening, including the Wassermann reaction and the Kahn test, and refuse those with a recent history of malaria. In areas where malaria is endemic presumably a negative film is deemed an adequate precaution.

## 21.6  Cardiac Arrest

Cardiac arrest has been recorded following rapid transfusion of more than 5 or 6 units of blood. Two factors have been held responsible:

1) Sodium citrate used to prevent clotting of transfused blood reduces ionised calcium which attaches itself to the citrate and becomes non-ionised. As ionic calcium is essential for cardiac systole, cardiac arrest may occur. Preventive measures are 5-10 ml intravenous calcium gluconate or calcium chloride whenever more than 4 units of blood have been infused. Recent investigations, however, have shown that although reduction in blood calcium does occur after repeated infusion of citrated blood, it is of short duration, because the liver and kidney rapidly remove the citrate from the body. Patients with depressed liver and kidney function, however, clear citrate more slowly, leaving low blood calcium, which could be regarded as a potential hazard.

2) An alternative theory accounts for cardiac arrest by hypothermia following rapid infusion of cold blood, which has been shown to be capable of reducing the oesophageal temperature to 29°C—a critical figure at which ventricular fibrillation can occur. To avoid cooling, steps are now taken to warm blood before infusion when large quantities are to be used, a practice which has reduced the incidence of ventricular arrhythmias and cardiac arrest during massive transfusions. There are two methods of warming blood. In one the blood passes through plastic coils immersed in a warm bath, and in the second the blood is passed through a microwave blood warmer. Microwave warmers are dangerous unless very carefully supervised; they can overheat and haemolyse the blood. A safer method is passage through plastic coils placed in a warm water-bath maintained at a constant temperature by a thermostat. The blood is maintained at 35°C, and no significant changes have occurred in the constitution of the blood, except for a slight rise in plasma haemoglobin concentration.

# 22 Recovery

## 22.1 Delegation of Responsibility

In law anaesthetists are responsible for their patients until they recover consciousness. To remain at the side of every anaesthetised patient until they were awake and responding would take up valuable operating time, so anaesthetists delegate responsibility for care during recovery to nurses or technicians. In order that anaesthetists can deal with an emergency complication, after their operation anaesthetised patients remain close to the operating theatre in a recovery room.

The delegation of responsibility for supervision of recovery of anaesthetised patients is in itself a hazard, but it is much reduced by good nursing and provision of essential equipment.

## 22.2 Equipment

Recently a hospital authority was criticised for failure to provide readily available equipment for cardiac resuscitation in a recovery room after a patient suffered severe brain damage following cardiac arrest. In addition, therefore, to a source of oxygen supply, suction apparatus, intravenous equipment, drugs, etc., every recovery room should include equipment for treatment of cardiac arrest (see Chap. 23), a sterile tracheostomy set, a mechanical ventilator (checked to be in working order every day) and monitoring equipment, central venous pressure lines and a 24-h service for blood gas analysis.

Fluorescent strip lighting is standard in new hospitals because it is economical and generates less heat than conventional lights. In recovery and anaesthesia areas, lights which give a blue tinge, suggesting the presence of cyanosis, should not be used. A shade known as 'warm white' is free from this objection.

## 22.3  Personnel

Nurses or technicians without experience (irrespective of seniority) should never be put in charge of a recovery room. Concentrating patients in recovery areas deprives ward nursing staff of experience in care of unconscious patients, and even senior staff should have a refresher course. A tragic accident occurred because a senior nurse unaccustomed to care of unconscious patients was put in charge of recovery.

One of the consultant anaesthetic staff should always be a member of the appointing committee selecting recovery room staff and should have the power to veto any candidate he or she thinks unsuitable.

## 22.4  Transfer of Patient to Recovery Room

When handing over the patient to recovery staff a full written account of the anaesthetic, of intravenous therapy and the cardiovascular state during the operation should be available, together with written instructions for postoperative care, including intravenous therapy and prescriptions for analgesic and anti-emetic medication. Unless there is a contra-indication, patients should always be nursed in the lateral position.

Before handing patients to recovery staff, anaesthetists should remove the endotracheal tube (if present) and ensure unobstructed respiration of normal amplitude, and that the circulatory condition is stable.

## 22.5  Removal of Endotracheal Tube

Before the tube is removed, a cough reflex must be present, the pharynx must be seen to be clear of blood and secretions and no residual paralysis must remain; residual paralysis would be shown by the presence of a 'tracheal tug' or by an inspiratory pause, indicating intercostal paralysis. If any blood is in the pharynx (e.g. after oral or ENT surgery) the patient should be turned on the side, the blood sucked out and the head lowered before removing the tube.

An airway of suitable size should be inserted into the mouth and the jaw drawn forward before withdrawing the tube. This is often accompanied by some coughing and laryngeal spasm, which soon subsides. Light manual pressure on a face-mask connected to a bag of oxygen helps the passage of oxygen into the lungs, should there be any spasm.

Exceptions exist to the above practice. After certain ophthalmic (see Chap. 38) and plastic procedures and operations to the head and neck (see Chap. 35) where coughing and spasm encourage haemorrhage and haematoma formation, anaesthesia should be deepened to minimise coughing on removal of the tube, but the patient should be put in the lateral position with head lowered.

## 22.6  Observation

Recovery room staff should maintain a record of progress in recovery using, if possible, the continuation of the anaesthetic record.

Oxygen administration is customary during recovery though some question its necessity in all patients.

Pulse, blood pressure and respiration of unconscious patients should be charted every 5-10 min, together with observations on the patient's general condition, for example whether the extremities are warm, dry and pink or cold, moist and cyanosed. Blood pressure measurement is unnecessary on conscious patients recovering from local anaesthetic blocks, besides being disturbing and mildly uncomfortable. If the pulse is palpable and the patient's condition satisfactory, the blood pressure assumes secondary importance.

Following application of plasters to arms and legs the limbs should be left open to view and inspected regularly to ensure the circulation is adequate.

## 22.7  Pain Relief

Anaesthetists should always chart an analgesic for pain relief and an anti-emetic. Failure results in unnecessary delay and distress to the patient whose memory of the painful episode remains long after everything else has been forgotten. After administration of an opiate, patients are usually kept in the recovery room for at least 30 min to exclude any untoward effects, e.g. vomiting or depression of respiration.

## 22.8 Complications

Complications related to the anaesthesia include depressed or obstructed respiration and certain cardiovascular effects; complications related to the surgery include external and internal haemorrhage and shock.

### 22.8.1 Respiratory Obstruction

The commonest cause of respiratory obstruction during recovery is the simplest to prevent, namely obstruction caused by the tongue falling into the pharynx. Partial obstruction is noisy and easy to detect. Total obstruction is silent, but efforts to breathe may be visible by retraction of the chest muscles and abdominal movement to depress the diaphragm. Covering the patient with blankets obscures this sign, but even when it is visible, an inexperienced observer could receive the impression that breathing was taking place. It is good practice for the chest and abdomen to remain visible until the swallowing reflex returns.

Obstruction can be completely avoided by turning unconscious patients into the lateral position before they leave the operating theatre. When that is not possible (after some orthopaedic and vascular operations), a recovery room nurse must hold the jaw forward and an oral airway be inserted and not removed until swallowing reflexes and muscle tone return.

Incomplete or partial obstruction from laryngeal spasm sometimes occurs after removal of the endotracheal tube. It is usually of short duration. The treatment of this condition has already been discussed in Sect. 12.3.1.

### 22.8.2 Respiratory Depression

Inadequate respiration can be of either central or peripheral origin. Inadequate respiration of central origin arises from depression by centrally acting opiate analgesics administered during the operation as part of the anaesthetic technique. Depression is obvious from the reduced rate and depth of breathing, associated sometimes with some degree of cyanosis. This last sign can be absent if the patient is breathing 100% oxygen.

Respiratory depression from opiates responds quickly to an intravenous injection of naloxone hydrochloride 0.4 mg in 2 ml or doxapram (Dopram) 20 mg in 5 ml. Although adequate respiration immediately follows intravenous injection, depression may recur owing to a cumulative effect of the opiates. This can be avoided if an intramuscular injection is given after the intravenous, thus prolonging its action.

Inadequate respiration also arises from muscular weakness due to inadequate elimination of muscle relaxant. Patients show a tracheal tug and breathing is laboured, with a pause after inspiration. Treatment of this condition has already been discussed in detail in Sect. 13.3.

### 22.8.3   Blood Pressure Changes

The significance of variations in blood pressure during recovery depends on the vasomotor tone or the critical closing pressure, which determines tissue perfusion, a vital concept when considering the significance of blood pressure changes during recovery.

Systolic blood pressure of less than 13.3 kPa during recovery is regarded by many as a hypotensive complication. Not everyone agrees. Provided perfusion is adequate, as shown by warm dry skin, dilated veins and an easily palpable pulse, no treatment is necessary.

Systolic pressures of around 10 kPa with all else normal require no treatment. Such figures are acceptable after spinal and epidural analgesia (see Sect. 17.3.1) and during induced hypotension (see Sect. 18.1.3) and sleep. Fears that the coronary circulation will become inadequate in elderly arteriosclerotic patients are ungrounded. Experimental work has shown that the percentage reduction of oxygen required by the heart during hypotension from lowered vasomotor tone exceeds the percentage fall in available oxygen from reduction in coronary flow. Therefore a net improvement of oxygen supply to the heart results.

Progressive fall in pressure, accompanied by a rising pulse rate and vasoconstriction, however, indicates an increase in vasomotor tone and rise of critical closing pressure due to sympathetic activity; perfusion becomes inadequate and cardiac output falls.

Some patients, especially those who recover quickly, have a normal or higher than normal blood pressure. Early return of pain sensation and sympathetic stimulation increases blood pressure. Complaint of pain calls for the injection of an opiate which, by reducing sympathetic activity, lowers blood pressure below pre-operative levels and does away with unnecessary anxiety.

Persistent hypertension is more dangerous and may indicate an undiagnosed phaeochromocytoma. Intravenous injection of 5 mg phentolamine (Rogitine) restores normal blood pressure. If hypertension persists, intravenous sodium nitroprusside (see Sect. 19.3) is effective and averts left ventricular failure.

### 22.8.4   Bradycardia

During recovery bradycardia can occur after spinal analgesia or halothane. It arises from increased vagal tone after reduction of sympathetic tone. The pulse rate increases as the anaesthetics wear off. If the pulse rate falls down lower than 50, restoration will follow an intravenous injection of 0.6-1.0 mg atropine.

### 22.8.5   External Haemorrhage

A wound dressing saturated with blood or excessive loss in the vacuum drains can draw attention to external haemorrhage. Blood loss in vacuum drains, e.g. after abdominoperineal operations or radical mastectomy, can often equal or exceed operative loss over a period of 12-24 h.

Haemorrhage from a tooth socket or after tonsillectomy is less obvious because the patient swallows the blood. But vomiting of clots will provide valuable clues.

The surgeon should be informed immediately. Until the surgeon arrives firm pressure is the correct treatment and, of course, continuation and speeding up of any intravenous fluids that are available. Bleeding tonsils or tooth sockets require general anaesthesia—a hazardous task (see Chap. 35).

### 22.8.6  Internal Haemorrhage

Progressive fall in blood pressure and rise in pulse rate, accompanied by pallor, sweating and restlessness, are signs of internal haemorrhage and shock. Treatment is discussed in Chap. 26. (N.B. In patients who have received chlorpromazine during anaesthesia or as sedation, signs of haemorrhagic shock are absent, except for a progressive fall in blood pressure, accompanied by pallor.)

### 22.8.7  Shock

Three types of shock may occur during recovery:

1) Shock ascribable to the operative procedure

2) Shock due to reactionary haemorrhage

3) Shock due to bacterial toxins, possibly exacerbated by over-enthusiastic administration of antibiotics.

*Operative Shock.* Signs of shock are not uncommonly seen in patients who have undergone major abdominal surgery. The shock is evident as constriction of veins on the back of the hand, pallor, and a bluish tinge around the lips and finger nails. Although the blood pressure is well maintained owing to vasoconstriction, the arterial oxygen tension is low and there is a rise in pulse rate. Inhalation of oxygen increases oxygen tension, but improvement is slow unless accompanied by intravenous administration of blood plasma or dextran.

A more severe shock may follow gall bladder or prostate surgery. It is characterised by more intense peripheral vasoconstriction and cyanosis, as well as a drop in blood pressure. Disturbances during surgery of old infected scar tissue release Gram-negative endotoxin into the bloodstream giving rise to Gram-negative shock. The condition responds to intravenous chlorpromazine 25 mg, provided a drip is still running.

*Haemorrhagic Shock.* Apart from reactionary haemorrhage, signs of haemorrhagic shock appear during recovery only if blood and fluid replacement has not been sufficient. If blood is not available, the loss must be replaced accurately with fresh frozen plasma, dried plasma, or dextran 70. If Hartmann's solution is used, a quantity double the calculated loss is necessary, since much of the solution enters the extracellular space.

Drug treatment and other aspects of shock are fully discussed in Chap. 26.

## 22.9 Return of Consciousness

The patient should remain in the recovery room until consciousness has returned and pulse, blood pressure and respiration remain stable for half an hour. Return of consciousness is preceded by return of muscle tone, particularly to the jaw and tongue muscles, and reappearance of swallowing reflexes, followed shortly by response to painful stimuli such as pinching an ear lobe or sternal pressure. Recovery is complete when patients respond to painful stimuli *and* to the spoken word, e.g. their name. Left undisturbed, many patients then fall asleep again, which is in many ways preferable to a restless recovery.

Factors affecting the rate of recovery are: (a) those related to physical state and susceptibility to premedicative and anaesthetic drugs, (b) pathological conditions of metabolic, endocrine and cardiovascular origin, (c) physiological disturbances, e.g. dehydration, metabolic acidosis and carbon dioxide retention.

### 22.9.1 Delay Due to Physical State

Frail, cachectic and elderly patients and those unaccustomed to alcohol are more susceptible to sedatives and anaesthetics of all sorts than normal subjects and may recover slowly. When dealing with such patients, it is best to avoid heavy sedative premedication and to use the minimum amount of intravenous induction agent, relying for the subsequent anaesthetic on inhalational agents, which enter and leave the body by a physical process through the lungs.

As pain contributes to recovery, delay often occurs after minor procedures (diagnostic endoscopies, ophthalmic surgery and minor gynaecological procedures), when postoperative pain is absent or slight.

### 22.9.2 Delay Due to Pathological Conditions

Liver disease, renal disease, diabetes, undiagnosed adrenal failure and cerebrovascular accidents may prolong recovery. Liver disease delays metabolism of barbiturates and prolongs the action of opiates. A small (50 mg) injection of pethidine to someone on the brink of liver failure can induce loss of consciousness. Renal disease delays the excretion of gallamine, which should not be used for such patients. Myxoedema (deficiency of thyroxine), diabetes, porphyria and muscular dystrophies are all associated with delay in recovery.

Sufferers from Addison's disease and patients with atrophied adrenals due to heavy steroid therapy may remain comatose unless they receive adequate steroid support (see Sect. 7.1). This possibility should be remembered when a patient remains unconscious, flaccid and with low blood pressure after a trivial surgical procedure.

Cerebrovascular disorders rarely delay recovery. Cerebral thrombosis, for example, delayed recovery only once in a series of 25 000 anaesthetics. The possibilities should be borne in mind when patients with head injuries do not recover.

### 22.9.3  Delay Due to Physiological Disturbances

Dehydration is theoretically a cause of delayed recovery but should be diagnosed during pre-operative assessment. Metabolic acidosis also causes delayed recovery (see Sect. 27.3.3).

Carbon dioxide retention is a cause of delayed recovery ($CO_2$ narcosis). During slow recovery from muscle relaxants, a low tidal volume does provide oxygen but is insufficient for elimination of carbon dioxide, so that the carbon dioxide concentration reaches narcotic concentrations.

Flushed skin and a bounding pulse are obvious aids to diagnosis. If blood gas analysis shows raised $P_{CO_2}$, treatment is simple and consists of performing mechanical ventilation through a soda lime canister to absorb the excess carbon dioxide. Treatment of delayed recovery from muscle relaxants is dealt with in detail in Sect. 13.3.2.

# 23 Cardiac Arrest

The possibility of cardiac arrest during anaesthesia can seldom be far from the mind of any working anaesthetist. Although the consequences of cardiac arrest can be devastating, to become obsessive and preoccupied with preventive measures carries a danger of lack of balance in anaesthetic techniques, and may lead to delay in preparation or denial of surgery to patients. The best insurance against cardiac arrest is observation of elementary rules, choice of the simple techniques and ensuring that the patient receives an adequate amount of the anaesthetic of choice.

## 23.1  Definition

Cardiac arrest can be defined as failure of cardiac contraction to deliver blood to the brain as a result of asystole or ventricular fibrillation. Diagnosis is made by absence of pulsation in a large artery, or sudden absence of bleeding during an operation. To wait for absence of a trace on a cardioscope can be misleading.

In unanaesthetised patients, loss of consciousness occurs, and, whether the patient is anaesthetised or not, respiration fails and the pupils dilate within 1 min. Death of nervous tissue occurs *on average* within 3 min. The precise time depends on the amount of oxygen in the body at the time. Complete recovery is more likely in those well oxygenated when arrest occurs. Where, however, oxygen lack is itself the cause of the arrest, the time available for full recovery is considerably less and although the heart's action may be restored, some degree of brain damage is inevitable.

## 23.2  Causes

Causes of cardiac arrest are legion. Those directly concerning anaesthetists are related to anaesthesia or surgery in operating theatres and recovery rooms, but arrests occurring anywhere in a hospital or clinic involve anaesthetists, who by reason of their special skills are always members of cardiac arrest teams.

### 23.2.1  During Anaesthesia and Recovery

Cardiac arrest during surgery has been estimated to occur in about 1:3000 operations. Regrettably, one quarter occur in the first few years of life, and two thirds in persons under the age of 50, many of whom appear to have been otherwise healthy.

Cardiac arrest during or immediately after anaesthesia and surgery may result from:

1) Technical errors
2) Anaesthetic agents and associated drugs
3) Pre-existing cardiac disease
4) Reflex stimulation
5) Surgical trauma, haemorrhage or air embolus
6) Airway obstruction

*Technical Errors.* Cardiac arrest during induction and maintenance of anaesthesia most commonly arises from failure of endotracheal intubation or, more rarely, from misuse of apparatus. Arrest during the recovery period is most often caused by obstructed airway, although secondary haemorrhage can also be a cause.

Errors of endotracheal intubation are discussed in Chap. 14 and the hazards from misuse of apparatus, faulty gas supplies, etc., in Chap. 10. Recovery room procedures and the hazards of respiratory obstruction are found in Chap. 22. No apology is needed for repeated mention of these hazards because such mistakes can be avoided by observing simple rules. Moreover, since oxygen lack is often the *cause*, some degree of brain damage is the rule and may be followed by expensive litigation.

*Anaesthetic Agents and Associated Drugs.* Overdose of anaesthetic agents rarely causes cardiac arrest unless patients are shocked, anaemic or cachectic. (The high mortality among shocked patients anaesthetised with large doses of thiopentone after the Pearl Harbor bombardment in 1942 is an example.)

The danger of cardiac arrest due to local analgesic agents and to surface application of cocaine after injection of local analgesic solutions containing adrenaline is mentioned in Chap. 17.

Adrenaline has been injected in mistake for atropine and caused arrest. All substances for injection should be carefully checked. Intra-arterial thiopentone has also caused arrest.

Induced hypotension can cause cardiac arrest, and ranks almost as high as obstructed airway or faulty apparatus as a causal factor, in the view of some insurance companies. Inexperience is the usual explanation.

Arrest from malignant hyperpyrexia (see Sect. 18.1.8) during anaesthesia is not associated with any specific agent. Hypothermia in patients who have received massive transfusions of unheated blood can also cause cardiac arrest (see Sect. 21.6).

*Pre-existing Cardiac Disease.* The hazards of anaesthesia with pre-existing cardiac disease are discussed in Chap. 2. The susceptibility of patients with 'fixed' cardiac output needs repeated emphasis. The susceptibility includes cases, for example, of aortic stenosis, aortic regurgitation and heart block (even with a pacemaker). Air embolus (see Sect. 21.4) is also a rare cause of cardiac arrest.

*Reflex Stimulation.* Enhanced vagal tone following stimulation of sensitive areas of lightly anaesthetised patients can cause bradycardia and arrest, for example during myringotomy, squint operations (oculo-cardiac reflex) or sudden dilation of the cervix.

*Surgical Trauma.* Trauma itself is not a cause of cardiac arrest, but association with severe haemorrhage is a possible factor. At the end of long operations requiring multiple transfusions, clotting deficiencies may occur, with massive haemorrhage which outstrips the rate of replacement.

*Airway Obstruction.* Obstructed airway has already been mentioned as the commonest cause of arrest in recovery areas.

### 23.2.2 Outside Operating Areas

The causes of arrest outside operating areas and recovery wards are too many to classify in detail and can only be listed. They comprise:

1) Disorders of heart muscle, especially occlusion of coronary arteries; myopathies; valvular disease, especially of the aortic valve, and Stokes-Adams syndrome (heart block, see Sect. 45.3).

2) Pulmonary embolus, which commonly occurs about the ninth day after major surgery, when patients are ambulant and prepared to depart for home

3) Compression of the heart by pericardial effusions with tamponade, e.g. following misplacement of a central venous pressure line (see Sect. 20.2)

4) Trauma, including rupture of the larger blood vessels and the heart in major accidents

### 23.3 Treatment

Treatment must begin as soon as arrest is diagnosed. During operations, absence of pulsation of a large artery is sufficient evidence. Restoration of oxygen supplies to the brain within 3 min is the first objective. Inflation of the lungs, either mouth to mouth or with oxygen by means of an automatically expanding bag, and external cardiac massage must start without delay.

Inflation of the lungs should continue through an endotracheal tube which should be passed as soon as possible. Cardiac massage should be continued externally, or internally if the abdomen is open. Internal massage is more effective than external massage.

Once oxygenation and some cerebral circulation is assured the cause—whether asytole or fibrillation—can be defined from an electrocardiogram tracing or by direct observation if the heart is visible.

Asystole should be treated by an intracardiac injection of 10 ml of 1% calcium chloride and/or 10 ml of a 1:10000 adrenaline solution, directly into the cavities of the heart. If calcium chloride does not succeed then adrenaline should follow immediately.

When, in the course of oxygenation, fibrillation changes from a feeble fine tremor to a coarse fibrillation, defibrillation can be attempted, preceded with advantage by intracardiac injection of 2 ml of 1:10000 adrenaline. The object of defibrillation is to pass an electric current through the heart, so that all fibres have a *simultaneous* refractory period, after which a normal beat should follow. Defibrillation may be by means of a direct current or an alternating current. Direct current is usually preferred. With the direct method, 15-100 W/s internally or 100-400 W/s externally causes less damage to cardiac muscle than the alternating current. For alternating current, 100-350 V internally, providing a current of 1-3.8 amp, or 300-750 V externally, providing a current of 3.8 amp, is passed initially for 0.2 s, but can be repeated at 0.5-s intervals if the first attempt is unsuccessful.

Once cardiac rhythm has been restored, steps should be taken to counteract acidosis by 8.4% sodium bicarbonate, and to reduce cerebral oedema by dehydrating solutions or dexamethasone (see Chap. 34).

The need for carefully written records of all the circumstances leading to a cardiac arrest and of the resuscitatory measures undertaken cannot be emphasised too strongly. An account made immediately after the incident, whilst memories are still clear, is an invaluable asset if, as often happens, allegations of negligence arise. In the absence of such adequate records these allegations are often difficult to refute.

# 24 Intensive Care

Special units designed for intensive care are a standard feature of any general hospital. Their primary function has been defined as treatment of acute illness, which, by intensive treatment, combined with unremitting and devoted nursing care, can restore many patients to an active life who in bygone years might not have survived.

The commonest conditions encountered in intensive care are respiratory, cardiac or renal failure and disturbances of electrolyte balance.

## 24.1 Administrative Responsibility

The frequent call for respiratory support and the special knowledge of such work which anaesthetists possess has meant they spend as much, if not more, time in intensive care units as renal, cardiovascular or respiratory physicians, who sometimes constitute the 'intensive care team'. For this reason anaesthetists often assume responsibility for the unit; this brings additional administrative hazards.

A major hazard to patients, and a source of frustration to nurses in intensive care, is conflicting advice received from a succession of consultants about treatment.

Some consultants prefer to retain control of treatment, although only visiting the unit once a day, when they sometimes countermand instructions dealing with specialised treatment (e.g. ventilation, dialysis) given by other experts, thus confusing nursing staff and upsetting patients.

This difficulty can be overcome by arranging that the resident doctor 'on call' for the unit is the only person to convey orders to nursing staff, thus avoiding conflicting orders. When differences occur, the resident can inform the consultants concerned and ask for guidance on the course to be adopted. Alternatively, in some units a multi-disciplinary approach exists, by which two or three consultants assume responsibility for all patients. Whilst this approach is administratively convenient, many younger consultants resent losing charge of patients at a critical stage.

## 24.2  Respiratory Distress and Mechanical Support

Conduct of mechnical ventilation, i.e. deciding when to start, how to maintain it and when to stop, is a main function of anaesthetists in intensive care units.

Several references have been made to the possible need for ventilator support by patients after major surgery (respiratory disease, prolonged action of relaxants, muscle dystrophies, thoracotomy, multiple rib fractures, etc.). It is not always easy to define the precise moment when mechanical assistance should begin. Started too soon, it may not be necessary, but it it is left too late, irreversible changes may occur.

In some units the decision to start mechanical ventilation is made after reference to the oxygen and carbon dioxide content of the blood and the patient's respiratory dynamics. Others base their decision on clinical assessment, a policy gaining in popularity; when carried out carefully, this gives better results than dependence solely on blood gas analysis. The details have been set out very clearly by Dr. A. Gilston in what he describes at the 'acute respiratory distress syndrome'.

The acute respiratory distress syndrome (ARDS) is a classical example of a vicious circle. Deterioration of lung function causes shortage of oxygen. Simultaneously, respiratory muscular effort increases, in an attempt to correct the deficiency of oxygen, but in so doing uses more, so that less is available for other vital areas, especially the brain and heart. Normally respiration at rest consumes about 3% of the total oxygen intake, but in patients with severe respiratory disease the proportion reaches 40%-50% of the total intake.

### 24.2.1  Evaluating respiratory distress
Respiratory distress can be evaluated by observation of the state of patients' respiratory, cardiovascular and central nervous systems and by assessing these signs by means of a simple scoring system which indicates need for ventilation.

*Respiratory Signs.* Breathlessness is a major sign and its intensity alone can determine the need for mechanical ventilation. Patients may deny *feeling* breathless, although it is obvious that talking itself presents difficulty because it uses up over 50% of the vital capacity.

*Facial Signs.* With increasing breathlessness the mouth remains constantly open, possibly in an effort to reduce airway resistance. Jerking of the tongue in the absence of curarisation is a bad prognostic sign.

Cyanosis or blueness of the lips is not as reliable as one would expect. Sufferers from cardiac disease or emphysema are often cyanosed at rest in the absence of any failure. On the other hand, the presence of cyanosed lips together with peripheral vascular failure and cold, clammy and cyanotic extremities, indicates shock and calls for immediate therapy (see Chap. 26).

Sweating of the forehead without peripheral cyanosis reflects increased respiratory muscular effort and not cabon dioxide retention. If, however, the skin is cold and clammy, there is need for intravenous supportive therapy.

The accessory muscles of respiration come into action in acute respiratory distress. The sternomastoid can be seen to be contracting forcibly and patients may even lift their heads off the pillow to increase this effect. On the other hand, movement of the alae nasi, a classical sign of great antiquity is not a particularly valuable sign and is less reliable than the open mouth.

*Neurological Signs.* As distress increases, consciousness deteriorates. The patient loses interest in surroundings and gazes vacantly ahead. Apathy slowly gives place to drowsiness and ultimately coma supervenes. Such changes have no relation to carbon dioxide or oxygen content of the blood and may occur whilst they are within normal limits.

The reasons for disturbance of consciousness are obscure. It often accompanies peripheral vascular failure and accompanying anoxia and its causes possibly are central and may arise from bacterial toxins or products of tissue degradation (the 'typhoid' state is an example).

*Cardiovascular Signs.* Peripheral circulatory failure becomes more evident with increasing respiratory distress. Pooling of blood in the capillary bed and falling cardiac output (as in shock) first become evident from cooling of toes and finger-tips, spreading later to the nose and ears. Standing at the end of a patient's bed feeling cold toes and observing an open mouth and breathlessness give sufficient evidence to justify immediate start of mechanical ventilation. Temperature changes can be shown more clearly by taking rectal and toe temperatures simultaneously. The difference between them becomes progressively greater as respiratory distress increases and diminishes again as the effects of treatment bring about an improvement.

Other cardiovascular signs include rising pulse, falling blood pressure, increase in central venous pressure and fall in urine output. The signs set out above are in many ways similar to those encountered in patients whose condition is deteriorating rapidly from bacterial shock. Recent experience in treatment of this condition has indeed shown that ARDS is a prominent feature and early installation of mechanical respiratory assistance causes a signficiant reduction in overall mortality.

*Scoring System for Acute Respiratory Distress Syndrome.* Assessment of the severity of the respiratory, cardiovascular and neurological signs included in the simple scoring system provides a reliable way of reaching a decision about the need to begin mechanical ventilation. If this is carried out carefully the resulting treatment is more effective than it would have been if the decision had been based on findings of blood gas analysis for their deterioration is often a late sign of respiratory distress.

The scoring system adopted selects common and important signs from the respiratory, cardiovascular and central nervous systems, omitting others, such as central venous pressure and oliguria, for simplicity. The selected signs are set out in Fig. 1.

| Resp. distress CVS CNS | | Dyspnoea, open, pursed, clenched lip biting, lip licking, cyanosis | | |
|---|---|---|---|---|
| Resp. system | Active alae nasi sweating | Dyspnoea, open, pursed, clenched lip biting, lip licking, cyanosis | | |
| C.V.S. | Cold | Cyanosis | Cold | |
| C.N.S. | Anxiety | Open | Response to nip | Apathy drowsiness |

**Fig. 1.** Selected signs of respiratory distress. Adapted from Gilston A (1976) Facial signs of respiratory distress after cardiac surgery: A plea for the clinical approach to mechanical ventilation Anaesthesia 31:385-397.

The respiratory signs in the scoring system are (a) activity of the alae nasi associated with sweating, (b) breathlessness, (c) an open mouth with the lips either pursed, or licking of the lips with the tongue.

The cardiovascular signs selected for inclusion in the scoring system are (a) a cold nose and cold extremities, (b) cyanosis of lips and nail beds, (c) a cold ear. Other cardiovascular signs which of course would influence decisions are, particularly, falling blood pressure and increase in pulse rate or arrythmias.

The neurological signs included are (a) anxious appearance, (b) apathy and drowsiness, (c) a poor or absent response to painful stimuli such as pinching the ear.

Mechanical ventilation should be initiated when the patient is breathless and shows two or more of the other signs listed above (cf. Fig. 2). Dr. Gilston's summary is worth quoting in full: 'Mechanical ventilation can be safely postponed if there are no cardiovascular signs provided respiratory distress is not severe and the patient is conscious, and if ventilation is immediately initiated when they appear.'

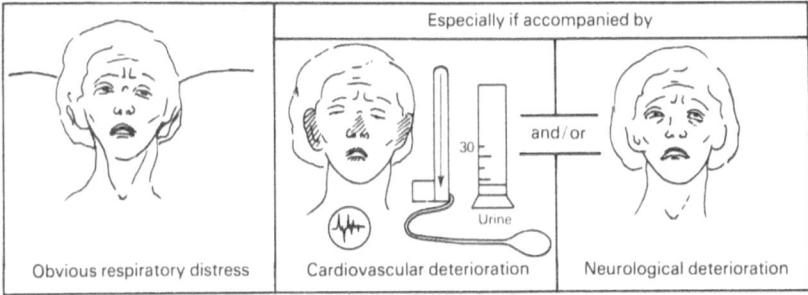

**Fig. 2.** Indications for ventilator treatment. Adapted from Gilston A (1976) Facial signs of respiratory distress after cardiac surgery: A plea for the clinical approach to mechanical ventilation. Anaesthesia 31:385-397.

The decision to start mechanical ventilation is purely arbitrary whatever the criteria, but the clinical approach has the merit of safety, simplicity and reliability and is readily learned. It only requires close observation and scrupulous care. A similar approach is required during weaning from the ventilator, which may be safely attempted without any tests of respiratory function if a patient is fully conscious, completely warm and the lungs clinically and radiologically satisfactory.

If there is any doubt, a delay of half an hour should precede a second examination. At this point it can often be seen whether vital signs have progressed or receded and whether new ones have appeared.

### 24.2.2 Mechanical Ventilation

The number of different ventilators increases yearly and appropriate textbooks and monographs should be consulted for details about their operation. The remarks in this chapter are for the benefit of those inexperienced in mechanical ventilation, who should use the same ventilator that they use for anaesthesia.

*Starting Ventilation.* If the patient is recovering from surgery and unconscious or partly conscious, mechanical ventilation with oxygen or air can start through an existing endotracheal tube with a tidal volume of 110 cm$^3$/kg, and a rate of 15-16 per minute. If a patient is conscious, initiation of ventilation may need light general anaesthesia with a relaxant to allow intubation, followed by hyperventilation with a carbon dioxide absorber, and as the effect of the relaxant wears off, intravenous injections of an opiate (pethidine 50-100 mg) to prevent 'fighting' the ventilator. After some hours, patients become more tolerant, being helped by intermittent administration of tranquillisers (phenothiazines, butyrophenones or diazepam). Otherwise paralysis with small doses of relaxants (5 mg pancuronium bromide) must continue.

*General Care.* Patients undergoing mechanical ventilation must *never* be left unattended. A sudden power failure can have fatal consequences and some alternative method must be available (e.g. Ambu bag) although most ventilators have a manual operative cycle.

*Communication.* Patients must always have paper and writing material and a bell to make their needs known. The presence of discomfort must be assessed and steps taken to relieve it. Restlessness, rising blood pressure and pulse rate are signs of inadequate ventilation.

*Tracheostomy.* If mechanical ventilation continues for more than 48 h, tracheostomy should be undertaken, improving the general comfort of the patient, easing swallowing and facilitating removal of secretions, whilst preventing laryngeal damage by the endotracheal tube. Tracheostomy should be carried out by a surgeon, so the details are not included here.

The main hazards of tracheostomy are infection and stenosis. Infection can be prevented by careful aseptic care of the wound. Dressings should be changed daily and a powerful antiseptic such as chlorhexidine used to cleanse it. Tracheal stenosis (the result of infection of the mucosa of the trachea) occurs in abou 3% of patients, but causes no symptoms unless the diameter is reduced by more than 60%. It can occur just above the stoma, at the site of the stoma, at the level of the tracheostomy cuff or just below it. The commonest sites are at the stoma itself, and at the level of the cuff.

Pressure of the cuff on the mucosa is a potential cause of mucosal damage, scar formation and contraction. The use of rubber has been abandoned in favour of plastic cuffs, the soft floppy type being the most suitable. Dilation to a pressure of about 1.5-2 kPa is enough for an airtight seal without damaging the tracheal epithelium.

*Suction.* The chief hazards of suction are introduction of infection from inadequate aseptic techniques and hypoxaemia from too early and too prolonged suction. Suction should be carried out with full aseptic technique. The catheter itself should be clipped or occluded until inserted to its full length, when it should be opened, suction taking place only during withdrawal, which should not be prolonged. The procedure can be repeated two or three times, provided it does not distress the patient.

*Humidification.* Water vapour and warmth must be added to inspired gases during mechanical ventilation because normal warming and humidification in passage through the nose and pharynx no longer operates. Failure to humidify inspired air results in drying the secretions in the trachea and bronchi; the secretions become tenacious, dried and crusty and impossible to remove. The simplest means of humidification is passage through a warm temperature-controlled water-bath.

*Physiotherapy.* The services of a physiotherapist experienced in care of patients on ventilators is essential since the physiotherapist's knowledge of ways and means of moving secretions is the key to successful treatment. Endotracheal suction alone is not sufficient to prevent accumulation of secretions from the deeper parts of the lung, whose periodic expansion is essential to prevent patchy areas of pulmonary collapse. Chest percussion during expiration following manual inflation of the lungs helps to mobilise secretions, but needs to be carried out by an expert. To be effective the treatment is often painful and exhausting, especially if a patient has multiple fractures of the ribs or sutured wound of chest or upper abdomen. Signs of distress are sweating and raised pulse rate. Some form of analgesia should be given—inhalation of nitrous oxide and oxygen or air and trichloroethylene, or intravenous opiates.

*Weaning.* When the reason for mechanical ventilation no longer exists, consideration must be given to weaning from the ventilator. Too sudden withdrawal upsets patients and they lose confidence. A normal chest X-ray should precede any attempt to wean the patient. At first, disconnection should only be for a short period, gradually increasing until the patient is off for an entire day. When confidence has increased, disconnection at night can start and then only if combined with sedation by tranquillisers that do not depress respiration.

## 24.3  Ethical Problems

Anaesthetists, especially those with administrative responsibilities in intensive care, may become involved in ethical problems concerning admission of hopeless cases, definition of brain death and its distinction from a vegetative state, and in dealing with potential donors of organs for transplantation.

### 24.3.1  Admissions
Intensive care units are basically intended for patients who have prospects of recovery and return to a reasonable existence. Hence terminal conditions are not usually admitted, and senile patients with terminal cardiorespiratory or cerebrovascular conditions have low priority. Attempts to predict the outcome for individual patients by computer are being undertaken but remain experimental.

### 24.3.2  Vegetative State
Survivors of acute brain damage who breathe spontaneously, but whose

cerebral cortex appears inactive, are said to be in a vegetative state. This state occurs after cardiac arrest associated with anoxia and after head injury. Because the brain stem remains active, sleep-wake rhythms remain and during waking time some minimal response to auditory or visual stimuli may be made, giving anxious relatives a false impression of returning consciousness. Once a vegetative state is established, intensive care has no more to offer and transfer to a unit for the long-term chronically sick should be arranged.

### 24.3.3 'Locked-in' Syndrome

A particularly tragic state results from total paralysis below midbrain level following thrombosis of basilar artery, polyneuritis, poliomyelitis, or myasthenia gravis. The cortex remains active and movements of eyes and eyelids may persist, allowing 'blinking' as the only means of communication with the outside world. Survival for long periods is possible with the aid of mechanical ventilation.

### 24.3.4 Brain Death

The vegetative state must be carefully distinguished from brain death, when ventilator support can justifiably be withdrawn, but sometimes not until after removal of kidneys or other organs for transplantation, for which the aid of anaesthetists is often sought. Brain death can be considered as a *possibility* when patients:

1) Are known to have irreversible brain damage

2) Are not breathing and have not received muscle relaxants or drugs which depress respiration

3) Are not hypothermic

Confirmation of brain death can be made on clinical grounds without EEG or cerebral angiography. Although EEG findings, if readily available, do offer moral support, if to procure such information means unnecessary delay it should not be sought because it prolongs the agony of waiting relatives.

The clinical criteria of brain death are:

1) Absence of all brain stem reflexes, including the pupillary, corneal, vestibulo-ocular, gagging and motor reflexes

2) Complete absence of breathing, established by disconnecting the ventilator and watching for return of spontaneous breathing as the blood carbon dioxide increases. This should take 5 min, provided the level of carbon dioxide was 5.3-6.1 kPa at the time of disconnection. If there are no facilities to measure plasma carbon dioxide, the patient should receive 5% carbon dioxide for 5 min *before* disconnection of the ventilator.

During disconnection, oxygen (6 litres/min) should be supplied by a tracheal catheter, which will provide adequate oxygenation by diffusion without increasing brain damage. Two examinations at 30-min intervals are essential and at least 6 h must have passed since the initial accident or admission to the unit.

### 24.3.5  Organ Transplantation

Before removal of organs for transplantation is to be considered, there are additional conditions to be met to conform with the Human Tissues Act:

1) Consent of next of kin must be obtained.

2) Two senior members of the hospital staff, not connected in any way with the transplant team, must agree in writing that diagnosis of brain death is completely justified.

Anaesthetists are often asked to keep patients oxygenated to ensure their optimum condition at removal of organs for transplantation. Two precautions are advised:

1) If not previously involved in the procedure of confirmation of brain death, the anaesthetist should disconnect the ventilator a third time, to obtain personal assurance that the diagnosis was correct and that the patient could not in any way be considered to be in a persistent vegetative state.

2) Although brain stem reflexes are absent in the damaged brain, spinal cord remains intact and reflex movements of limbs can occur in response to surgical stimuli, for example after incision of the skin. Such movement causes considerable emotional disturbance amongst assisting nursing and technical staff and can be avoided by giving a paralysing dose of a muscle relaxant, which masks any remaining activity of the spinal cord.

# Part III

*Emergency Surgery*

# 25 Stomach Content

Emergency conditions requiring anaesthesia arise from domestic, industrial or road traffic accidents and from acute abdominal conditions. The associated anaesthetic hazards do not always bear a direct relationship to the seriousness of the surgical problem and all share one common major hazard, stomach content, which may consist of an undigested meal, of blood and clots, or of a dark brown fluid—the 'coffee-ground' vomit of intestinal obstruction.

Undigested food is often present in the stomach of victims of domestic or road traffic accidents. Although the normal emptying time is 3 h, delay invariably occurs after accidents because of gastric stasis due to sympathetic activity, to which pain, anxiety and pain-killing opiates contribute.

If enquiry elicits information about a recent meal or liquid refreshment, delay of 5 h should take place, unless the emergency operation is of a life-saving nature. Metoclopramide (Maxolon) 26 mg intravenously is said to increase the speed of gastric emptying, but should not alter the 5-h rule. A sophisticated way of ensuring an empty stomach is to give the patient a barium swallow and X-ray the stomach every half-hour, until all barium has passed from the stomach and can be seen to have entered the small intestine.

Gastric contents are also present in acute abdominal emergencies. Although the presence of blood or coffee-ground vomit is obvious in most acute abdominal conditions, it sometimes may only be revealed by inquiry. Even patients with large-bowel obstruction may not admit to vomiting, although the stomach is full of coffee-ground vomit.

## 25.1  Dangers

A full stomach from any cause is a hazard during induction and maintenance of anaesthesia since, should the contents well up into the pharynx, cardiac arrest can occur from anoxia due to obstruction by undigested food, or massive inhalation into the lungs. Inhalation of smaller amounts, whilst not fatal, can cause pneumonitis and collapse of the lung, which are not always evident until the appearance of cyanosis and breathlessness during recovery. Lung abscess may also be a late results.

## 25.2 Vomiting and Regurgitation

Stomach content can reach the pharynx as the result either of vomiting (an active process), or of regurgitation (a passive process). The distinction between the two is not always appreciated, and often what is described as vomiting is in fact regurgitation.

Vomiting is a reflex act of considerable complexity involving both autonomic and somatic nervous systems. Simultaneous salivation, bradycardia, reverse peristalsis, and inhibition of respiration requires a degree of nervous integration not possible in anaesthetised subjects. When vomiting occurs, laryngeal reflexes remain fully operative and if patients are immediately put into the lateral position with a head-down tilt and steps taken to clear the pharynx by suction or manual removal of solid vomit, catastrophes can be avoided.

Regurgitation of stomach content is a passive, silent process and a special danger in unconscious patients, whose laryngeal reflexes have been rendered useless through the paralysis induced by muscle relaxants. Regurgitation however will not occur in such patients unless the intra-gastric pressure rises from the normal 0.5-0.7 kPa to 1.8 kPa or higher.

## 25.3 Anaesthetic Techniques

Junior anaesthetists are often asked to induce anaesthesia in accident and emergency departments for reduction of dislocations or fractures or for sutures of lacerations. The request often comes casually, for a 'whiff of gas' or a 'shot of Pentothal'. The procedures are often not as short as suggested, nor are they free from anaesthetic complications arising from a full stomach.

### 25.3.1 Local Analgesia

Before considering a general anaesthetic in such circumstances, careful consideration must be given to the use of regional methods. These should be used whenever possible, as they are ideal ways of overcoming the problems associated with stomach contents.

Most lacerated wounds can be dealt with by local infiltration or regional block. Fractures and dislocations of the upper limb can often be treated by brachial plexus block, and forearm and hand injuries by intravenous lignocaine (see Chap. 17).

Spinal or epidural methods are ideal for surgery of the lower extremities and abdomen, provided that any shock, dehydration, disturbed acid-base balance, etc., have received adequate treatment. Strangulated inguinal or femoral hernias can also be treated by a local block, if epidural or subdural methods are thought unsuitable.

### 25.3.2 General Anaesthesia

Before contemplating anaesthesia for any emergency condition, anaesthetists should always enquire the time and constituents of the last meal taken, and of any liquid refreshment taken subsequently. A patient admitted to hospital after a road traffic accident at 11 p.m. may admit to having eaten a meal at 6 p.m., but unless questioned may not add that in the ensuing hours considerable quantities of liquids were taken. This information must be recorded, as it has considerable medical and legal importance.

*Equipment.* Anaesthesia for patients with suspected stomach contents should never be undertaken without a tipping-table, suction apparatus in working order and the assistance of a technician or nurse with training and experience in emergencies. An accident room without these things is not a suitable place to anaesthetise patients suspected of having a full stomach.

*Measures to Empty a Full Stomach.* Passage of a number 6 nasogastric tube with the patient in the lateral position allows aspiration of stomach contents if they are clear and not too thick. Attempts at passing a gastric tube may induce vomiting and thus empty the stomach. Although unpleasant for the patient, vomiting in this position is safe, as the vomited matter runs out of the mouth, automatically disposing of a serious hazard.

If blood or viscous matter is in the stomach a larger, size 12 tube should be passed through a previously cocainised nostril to the stomach. This allows aspiration of blood and viscous matter. However, many advise that the tube should be withdrawn before induction, because it interferes with the integrity of the cardio-oesophageal sphincter.

*Premedication.* In emergency, premedication should be confined to atropine, which in addition to its well known drying properties, also increases cardio-oesophageal tone and reduces the likelihood of regurgitation.

*Inhalational Induction.* When presence of gastric contents is suspected, inexperienced anaesthetists should avoid intravenous induction and depend on an inhalational technique with which they are familiar.

Before induction a slight head-down tilt should be chosen and the patient turned into the lateral position. Induction can be either with halothane and oxygen or with cyclopropane and oxygen. Both these agents ensure rapid induction of anaesthesia without coughing and spasm, taking the patient rapidly down to the first plane, third stage, of anaesthesia. If the second plane, third stage, has been used the patient can safely be turned into the supine position, and intubation can usually be performed without muscle relaxants, although the vocal cords do remain active and will close if the endotracheal tube touches them.

Methods similar to the above were routine in pre-relaxant days and even after the introduction of relaxants. Many senior and much respected anaesthetists felt safer with this method. They argued that laryngeal, tracheal and bronchial reflexes remained active and intubation was quite practicable before their total abolition. They felt that paralysis by muscle relaxants *before* insertion of an endotracheal tube exposed the patients to unjustifiable risks from inhalation of regurgitated stomach content.

*Intravenous Induction.* The preliminaries should be as for inhalational methods and if an intravenous drip has not been set up some form of indwelling needle should be put in place. The choice of intravenous agent is not of great significance.

Reference has already been made to the danger of muscle fasciculation after suxamethonium causing reflux into the pharynx from the increased intragastric pressure. Those who use this relaxant always make sure an assistant is present to exert pressure on the cricoid (Sellick's manoeuvre). If rapid relaxation is wanted, the new non-depolarising agent fazadinium is preferable.

If difficulties are encountered during intubation, a careful watch should be kept for signs of returning muscle activity, for this also means the laryngeal reflexes are returning, and with lightening intravenous anaesthesia a danger of laryngospasm arises. Attempts at intubation should be halted and the patient allowed to inhale a mixture of oxygen and anaesthetic vapour until injection of additional muscle relaxant has produced further relaxation. In this way anaesthetists can prevent regurgitation of small amounts of gastric contents during spasmodic expulsive movements.

# 26 Shock: Vascular Responses to Injury, Haemorrhage and Infection

Shock, whether traumatic, haemorrhagic or bacterial, constitutes an ever-present hazard for anaesthetists. Its occurrence is always a possibility during or immediately after major surgical operations, whilst its actual presence very often coincides with emergency conditions. If undetected and not treated it adds greatly to the hazards of emergency anaesthesia, a consideration which justifies its inclusion at this point.

## 26.1 Definitions

The word 'shock' is widely used to describe several different conditions associated with collapse. Thus there is neurogenic shock (fainting or vasovagal attacks), anaphylactic shock (sensitivity to foreign proteins) and electric shock, but the clinical manifestations of these conditions do not have much in common.

There is also shock of cardiac, bacterial, haemorrhagic and traumatic origins; these are often described and treated as separate entities but their clinical signs have a great deal in common.

Use of the term 'shock' in clinical discussion will probably continue for many years because everybody concerned knows what it means, although those who devote their entire time to its study prefer to talk and think about 'response to injury', which they subdivide into neuro-endocrine, metabolic, cardiorespiratory and reticulo-endothelial.

All patients undergoing surgical operations are injured and the nature of their responses determines the subsequent clinical course. Anaesthesia plays a much greater part than is generally appreciated in regulating response to injury, a function that is as important as pain suppression. For example, the introduction of chloroform anaesthesia halved the mortality of mid-thigh amputation, showing how even a crude method of anaesthesia can reduce response to injury.

Although response to injury occurs in all operated patients, no one mentions 'shock' until the cardiovascular response can be seen and measured.

## 26.2  Neural Basis

Successful treatment of any medical condition is impossible without a knowledge of the underlying physiological and pathological disturbances. The greater the number of cures recommended for any medical condition, the less one discovers is known about its actual cause.

Successful treatment of shock is also not possible without some idea of its physiology and pathology, which would then suggest what type of therapy might be effective in its prevention or reversal.

Although textbooks classify causes of shock, few explain why so many different factors produce virtually the same syndrome. Participation of the central nervous system in these processes could provide an answer.

An impressive amount of high quality modern research supports the concept (put forward half a century ago by Crile) that response to injury is a function of the central nervous system and that the integrative centre is the hypothalamus. The same sources also confirm a long-standing idea of close involvement of the sympathetic nervous system. A concept conferring a widespread integrative function on the hypothalamus as well as an intimate relationship with the sympathetic nervous system becomes more credible after a brief survey of its afferent and efferent connections.

On the afferent side a formidable amount of information from somatosensory and autonomic sources reaches the hypothalamus via the pontomedullary reticular formation. The intricate cellular arrangement of the reticular formation is slowly being unravelled. Cellular variety is infinite and axons, far from being short as originally suggested, extend upwards and downwards with a multiplicity of interconnections.

One authority has estimated that one reticular cell and its dendrites have a potential for interaction with 4000 other cells, and that if one includes axons and their collaterals, the figure reaches 27 000 cells. Furthermore, axons from reticular cells have been shown to reach the hypothalamus via the posterior longitudinal bundle and the limbic system and fornix.

A prominent feature of reticular neurones is the non-specificity of their response to external stimuli of widely differing origin. Micro-electrode studies have shown that one reticular neurone will respond at different times to stimuli of fore or hind legs (somatic nervous system) as well as to stimuli of the nose or the ear (5th and 8th cranial nerves). This property has led some authorities to describe the reticular formation as the 'non-specific nervous system'.

Although it is well known that the reticular formation controls wakefulness and muscle tone, its capacity to affect vasomotor, respiratory and endocrine activity in response to external stimuli is less widely appreciated. These activities together with its rich somatic and autonomic afferent connections and the non-specificity of the response of its neurones provide a credible hypothetical arrangement for regulation of changes in the internal or external environment.

The participation of the sympathetic nervous system in the peripheral response to injury has already been mentioned. The knowledge that the reticular formation contains an extensive noradrenergic neuronal system provides one more link in the chain of evidence for participation of the central nervous system in the response to injury.

In brief, a collection of noradrenergic neurones in the locus ceruleus of the pontomedullary reticular formation send axons upwards to the hypothalamus and downwards to the lateral sympathetic outflow of the spinal cord. During experimental haemorrhagic and traumatic shock an increase in noradrenaline turnover takes place in the hypothalamus and noradrenergic neurones in the hypothalamus examined after death from irreversibility show evidence of damage.

Noradrenergic neurones, through their connections with the lateral sympathetic outflow, can initiate discharge from sympathetic ganglia, whose efferent fibres expand as varicosities around the terminal arterioles, their noradrenaline content being 600 times that of the parent cell.

As walls of the terminal arterioles are almost entirely smooth muscle, the effect of a strong sympathetic discharge upon them has been aptly described as 'sphincteritic' in nature, and could account for the severe vasospasm seen in severe shock.

Although circulatory changes have received emphasis because they can be seen and their effects to some extent measured by anaesthetists, metabolic, endocrine and reticulo-endothelial responses share equal significance and are regulated through hypothalamic activity.

There is evidence that reticulo-endothelial responses are the consequences of sympathetic nervous action and that endocrine responses arise through the neurohypophysis. For example, activity in the supraoptic nucleus of the hypothalamus stimulates release of pitressin (ADH) which converts angiotensin I to angiotensin II, stimulating release of noradrenaline, whose action pitressin itself intensifies, compromising the renal circulation and to a less extent that of the lungs and liver.

Centrally induced sympathetic activity in response to injury is evident as vasoconstriction affecting both arteriolar and venous systems. The greatest intensity occurs in mesenteric, renal, hepatic, pulmonary, cutaneous and muscular vascular systems, making more blood available for the heart and central nervous system vessels, which are less affected. Vasoconstriction results in 'ischaemic anoxia', which persists for 2 or 3 h before deteriorating into 'stagnant anoxia'. Arteriolar dilatation replaces constriction, but since constriction of small venules persists, blood cannot return to the general circulation and accumulates in the capillary bed.

Progressive oxygen lack increases capillary permeability, so that serum and later red and white blood cells pass into the interstitial tissues, leading subsequently to widespread haemorrhage and infarct formation, described as circulatory decay, with all the features of disseminated intravascular coagulation.

Such basic circulatory changes occur whether the shock is traumatic, haemorrhagic, bacterial or cardiac in origin. They differ only in intensity, being far more severe in bacterial shock, since bacterial toxins have such a strong (though little appreciated) affinity for sympathetic nervous tissue, including that in the central nervous system, that a state of stagnant anoxia exists from the start.

### 26.3 Diagnosis and Treatment

The clinical signs of shock arise from poor perfusion, the result of vasoconstriction. They include pallor, sweating, a cyanotic tinge to lips and nail beds and a progressive fall in blood pressure and rise in pulse rate. Temperature regulation is disturbed. Skin temperature becomes subnormal and rectal temperature rises. Patients complain of feeling cold and may shiver. A nose that is cold to the back of the hand is a well known sign of shock.

Restlessness is common after severe haemorrhage; respiration may become gasping owing to acute oxygen lack, a sign known as 'air hunger'.

The transition to stagnant anoxia is accompanied by deterioration of renal, pulmonary and gastro-intestinal function. Renal disorder is indicated by reduced urinary output, albuminuria and a raised blood creatinine, pulmonary disorder by hyperventilation, dyspnoea and a low plasma oxygen, whilst haemorrhage and ileus indicate involvement of the gastro-intestinal tract.

The idea that all types of shock are the consequence of the impact of nervous impulses entering the central nervous system from different sources, but which activate the same nervous pathways in the reticular formation, simplifies the approach to treatment. Basic principles, apart from removal of the cause, should not differ; they comprise relief of vasospasm and restoration of normal tissue perfusion.

In many instances intelligent anticipation can prevent the more serious signs of shock, especially from haemorrhage or trauma. Disposable plastic equipment, particularly intravenous cannulae, have made intravenous therapy a routine procedure for most injured patients admitted to accident and emergency departments, so that haemorrhagic and traumatic shock are rare.

### 26.3.1 Haemorrhagic Shock

Notwithstanding the above, haemorrhagic shock may still follow acute haemorrhage after peptic ulceration, ruptured ectopic gestation, ruptured abdominal aneurysm, or traumatic rupture of liver or spleen. The signs of shock are usually present and conventional treatment is with opiates, to alleviate pain and anxiety, and vigorous transfusion of fresh frozen plasma, or plasma expanders, under pressure if necessary, until cross-matched blood becomes available. Surgery can begin when a recordable blood pressure is present, for perfusion always improves after inhalation of low concentrations of halothane.

Haemorrhagic shock occasionally occurs during radical surgery for malignant disease, for example bladder tumours previously treated by radiotherapy. Unobserved suction can lead to errors in estimation of blood loss unless anaesthetists ask for regular reports on the contents of suction bottles, if the latter are concealed by instrument tables, etc.

After sudden severe haemorrhage during an operation a catastrophic fall in blood pressure can occur. The patient should be immediately put in a steep head-down tilt and the surgeon asked to pack the wound and stop operating until rapid infusion, under pressure, of blood, plasma or plasma expanders restores peripheral circulation and blood pressure becomes recordable.

### 26.3.2 Traumatic Shock

Traumatic shock is more severe than haemorrhagic shock, which is often also present but, being internal, not always recognised until after failure of preliminary resuscitatory measures.

A relationship has been observed between the swelling seen round fractured bones and reduction in blood volume, which was said to represent extravasated blood, requiring replacement by transfusion. Open operations for fractured bones do not reveal extravasated blood, the swelling consisting of oedematous muscle and clear serous fluid.

Blood volume studies in injured patients are unreliable because of wide variations in normal blood volumes, and because the dye dilution method with which these studies were made only measures circulating blood volume, omitting blood incarcerated in the capillary bed owing to shock.

Treatment of traumatic shock does not differ from that of haemorrhagic shock, and is by intravenous fluids and blood when available. Since pain and anxiety contribute to its severity, opiates and tranquillising agents should be prescribed. Blood is not essential except when haemorrhage is present. Failure to respond to simple measures should arouse suspicion (as already indicated) of internal injuries and haemorrhage.

### 26.3.3  Gram-negative Shock

In the 1950s reports appeared of a syndrome associated with Gram-negative bacteraemia in surgical patients which became known as Gram-negative shock. An immense literature has accumulated about this condition, whose mortality remains in the region of 50% in spite of the availability of antibiotics capable of freeing the blood stream of Gram-negative organisms. That a similar syndrome occurs in patients dying from typhoid fever (also a Gram-negative infection) seems to have escaped the notice of those concerned with this condition. A possible explanation is that treatment of typhoid is so successful with antibiotics that patients seldom die.

Failure to appreciate this has led to much misunderstanding about the condition. Gram-negative shock does not differ from bacterial shock caused by Gram-positive organisms, which also has been virtually eliminated by antibiotic therapy.

Gram-positive organisms produce an exotoxin, so that their pathological effects cease when they are destroyed. The reverse is true for Gram-negative infections, whose pathological effects arise from the endotoxin released by them when they are destroyed. Patients with a Gram-negative bacteraemia often remain ambulant, e.g. in the early stages of typhoid, and only become ill when immune responses and/or antibiotics destroy the organisms releasing endotoxin into the bloodstream.

When the endotoxin reaches the central nervous system, it causes severe signs of Gram-negative shock through its affinity for and irritant action on noradrenergic nervous tissue in the brain stem; this action is five hundred times as strong as that resulting from action on peripheral sympathetic nerve endings.

For this reason a cautious approach to antibiotic therapy is advisable, in order to avoid release of too much endotoxin at any one time. 'Loading' doses should be avoided and modest doses of antibiotics prescribed, patients being examined at regular intervals for any signs of toxicity. Danger signs include a sudden fall in temperature and blood pressure, with tachycardia, pallor and cyanosis of the extremities; reduction of urinary output accompanied by haematuria and albuminuria; and raised blood creatinine. Appearance of any of the above should be an indication for withholding antibiotic therapy until supportive treatment has restored the peripheral circulation. The adoption of such a regime in treating typhoid patients with bacteraemia some years ago prevented sudden collapse and death in typical Gram-negative shock during antibiotic therapy and reduced the mortality from between 12% and 15% to zero.

These considerations do not apply to antibiotic treatment of Gram-negative intestinal or urinary tract infections, where the endotoxin produced by destruction of Gram-negative organisms passes out in the urine or faeces, producing only localised areas of ischaemia with sloughing and ulceration, and conceivably accounts for antibiotic-related colitis.

## 26.4  Drug Therapy

Many therapeutic agents have been used to prevent or treat shock states, mostly with little success. They include cardiac and circulatory stimulants; adrenolytic agents; deafferentation of the central nervous system; and hydrocortisone.

### 26.4.1  Cardiac and Circulatory Stimulants

Depressed circulation, low blood pressure and poor cardiac output encouraged trial of vasopressors and cardiac stimulants in the treatment of shock, but without success. The failure is not surprising, since vasopressors intensify vasoconstriction, and adrenaline is capable of inducing shock in dogs.

The most successful cardiac stimulant has been isoprenaline, an inotropic and beta-sympathomimetic agent that vasodilates muscles, and increases the strength and rate of the heart beat.

### 26.4.2  Adrenolytic Agents

Increased appreciation of the part played by overactivity of the sympathetic nervous system in the development of shock has led to the use of adrenolytic substances in its prevention and treatment.

The object is to prevent vasoconstriction either by blockade of sympathetic ganglia or by interference with noradrenaline at sympathetic nerve endings. There are reports that dibenzyline is of value in Gram-negative shock, and ganglion blockers and sodium nitroprusside in haemorrhagic shock. Alpha and beta blockade has not met with success. Although adrenolysis is a logical approach, total chemical sympathectomy increases rather than decreases mortality of experimental tourniquet shock.

### 26.4.3  Deafferentation

An alternative approach, especially attractive to those who advocate a neural basis for shock, is to consider ways of reducing the impact of incoming stimuli on the central nervous system by a process of deafferentation.

Shock *prevention* through deafferentation by subdural and epidural blockade is an established fact, but these methods are of no value for treating shock, once present, either in experimental animals or in clinical practice.

Chlorpromazine, effective in prevention of haemorrhagic and bacterial shock, has established deafferenting properties. Its adrenolytic action is incorrectly regarded as arising from alpha and beta blockade, although several years ago its vasodilator action was shown in human subjects to be central rather than peripheral in origin. More recent neruophysiological research has shown that it reduces the effect of peripheral stimuli on the reticular formation at the point where sensory collaterals synapse with reticular neurones through an antagonistic action on the excitatory effects of noradrenaline.

The anaesthetic literature over the past 20 years has contained several references, from many parts of the world, to the value of chlorpromazine in preventing and treating shock states. Since much misunderstanding exists about the action of chlorpromazine, the following facts should be borne in mind when prescribing it for patients.

Chlorpromazine opens up the circulation by a vasodilator action which virtually abolishes the vasoconstrictor reflex response to haemorrhage. It should never be given intravenously if vasoconstriction is evident, unless an intravenous infusion has been set up to fill up the dilated vessels (and then only in 5-mg doses), the motto being, 'Open up and fill up'. However, if vasoconstriction makes vein puncture difficult, a small intramuscular dose of about 25 mg chlorpromazine produces sufficient vasodilation to facilitate vein puncture without a dangerous fall in blood pressure.

Intravenous chlorpromazine often causes a tachycardia, possibly through a reflex from an irritant effect on veins. It does not occur when diluted in 1 litre of saline, and is much reduced if intravenous injection is preceded by an intramuscular dose an hour or so beforehand. The tachycardia is harmless and usually settles within 24 h.

Chlorpromazine reduces vasomotor tone, lowers critical closing pressure (see Chap. 20) and thus reduces systolic blood pressure. Provided patients are not hypovolaemic, no harm results. The hypotension resembles that occurring from partial deafferentation during normal sleep and even a mild surgical stimulus immediately restores the pressure to near normal figures.

Jaundice, sometimes obstructive, occurs in psychiatric patients who consume large oral doses of chlorpromazine. It is the result of hypersensitivity of the cells of the bile canaliculi which swell and obstruct the flow of bile. A minimum of 5 days' oral consumption is necessary for development of hypersensitivity. In over 25 years' regular use of chlorpromazine, administering it both intramuscularly and intravenously, the author has never encountered jaundice as a sequela.

The deafferenting properties of chlorpromazine reduce the alerting action of sensory input on the reticular formation and make the central nervous system more susceptible to all central depressant drugs, the doses of which can therefore be significantly reduced. If given in the course of a normal anaesthetic, recovery time will be considerably prolonged. The shock-preventing properties of chlorpromazine being better than its curative properties, it should be administered as early as possible, as a preventive measure, in situations where shock is likely to develop.

*Traumatic Shock.* On admission to accident and emergency departments, all injured patients should receive an intramuscular injection of 50 mg chlorpromazine and 50-100 mg pethidine, and an intravenous infusion. Even though signs of shock are not present on admission, many patients, after an hour in the X-ray department without any treatment, return to the accident and emergency department showing signs of traumatic shock, requiring resuscitation before anaesthesia and surgery. Patients receiving chlorpromazine do not require resuscitation and have an excellent urinary output. The combination of an analgesic and a tranquillising action relieves pain and reduces anxiety, both of which are contributory factors to shock states.

*Haemorrhagic Shock.* Patients with acute gastro-intestinal haemorrhage often show signs of shock, particularly in the form of venospasm, which slows up and even stops intravenous infusions. Although hypotensive, such patients respond favourably to 5-mg doses of chlorpromazine at 5-min intervals until not more than 25 mg has been given. Usually vein spasm disappears after 10-15 mg, as is evident from the speeding up of the infusion and improvement in pulse pressure. Rapid infusion of blood should continue until the blood pressure returns to the pre-operative levels. In one published series this routine reduced mortality by 15%. Urine output in the patients so treated exceeded 1 litre in 24 h, compared with an average of 300 ml in a control series.

*Operative Shock During Surgery.* The use of chlorpromazine to treat operative shock, especially during *surgical* operations is dangerous. Although blood replacement may appear adequate, administration of chlorpromazine may result in severe falls in blood pressure, requiring treatment by head-down tilt and rapid infusion under pressure. The reason is that vasoconstriction is often more widespread than appears from observation and hence the effects of opening up the circulation are more severe than expected. A better plan is to include chlorpromazine in the anaesthetic technique in anticipation of possible operative shock, a policy which takes full advantage of its preventive properties.

*Postoperative Shock.* From time to time patients recovering from upper abdominal and gall bladder surgery, especially, show signs of shock, pallor, cyanosed and cold extremities, and hypotension with reduced $Pa_{O_2}$ which does not readily respond to oxygen and intravenous therapy.

Treatment with intermittent 5-mg intravenous injection of chlorpromazine in saline reverses cyanosis and restores normal blood oxygen tension and systolic blood pressure.

*Bacterial or Endotoxin Shock.* Both chlorpromazine and hydrocortisone can prevent experimental endotoxin shock, but their curative action is less pronounced.

Nevertheless intravenous chlorpromazine is capable of reversing endotoxin shock if given early, before signs associated with stagnant anoxia (renal and respiratory failure) are present. Signs of respiratory distress syndrome (see Sect. 24.2) are indications for mechanical support of ventilation, which, when instituted early, has been shown to reduce mortality.

As already mentioned, antibiotic therapy, if administered too freely, can intensify Gram-negative shock. Since the preventive properties of chlorpromazine (and hydrocortisone) are superior to their curative properties, it seems sensible to administer these agents, together with antibiotics, to patients with known or suspected Gram-negative bacteraemia, rather than wait until the signs of shock appear before giving them. There appears no point in prescribing antibiotic therapy to patients already showing clinical signs of endotoxin shock, until intravenous therapy, oxygen and hydrocortisone or chlorpromazine have restored peripheral circulation and renal function. Such a policy may appear heretical but, as already mentioned, it has been applied with success in the treatment of typhoid fever. Furthermore, there is no evidence that antibiotics, although sterilising the bloodstream, have made any contribution to reducing mortality from this disastrous complication, which still remains in the region of 50%.

Renal failure associated with depressed liver function arises from the inability of the liver to detoxify endotoxins, which accumulate in the bloodstream causing renal vasoconstriction and failure. The only prospect of any success lies in attempting to reverse shock and improve perfusion, particularly of the liver, with either hydrocortisone or chlorpromazine and intravenous infusion.

A worker in Scandinavia treats patients with shock failing to respond to conventional therapy in a constant-temperature environment. Intermittent injections of 5 mg chlorpromazine with intravenous infusion raise the lowered skin temperature and reduce the raised rectal temperature. When the two temperatures become equal, peripheral perfusion has been restored and shock reversed.

# 27 Disturbances of Fluid, Electrolytes and Acid-Base Balance

## 27.1  Dehydration

One should suspect dehydration if there is a history of vomiting and diarrhoea or of inadequate intake of fluid, due for example to oesophageal stricture or simply weakness. Dehydrated patients have a dry, furred tongue, wrinkled inelastic skin, sunken eyeballs and prominent cheek bones. Urine output is reduced, very concentrated and, when salt depletion exists, contains no chloride.

Simple water deficiency should be distinguished from salt depletion by the history of the condition. Water depletion (due to the patient being unable to swallow or too weak to take fluid) is best treated by 5% dextrose until clinical improvement occurs and flow of urine takes place. Reduction of haemoconcentration as shown by repeated haematocrit estimations indicates the effectiveness of treatment.

## 27.2  Electrolyte Deficiencies

Salt depletion is usually accompanied by deficiencies in potassium, copper, phosphate and magnesium. When facilities are available, blood should be taken for estimation of all electrolytes, pH and base excess at the beginning of treatment with intravenous fluids.

*Treatment.* The fluid choice is Hartmann's solution or Ringer lactate, which is isotonic, and whose chloride content (0.6%) equals that of the extracellular fluid. It also contains a bicarbonate precursor in the form of sodium lactate and a trace of potassium. One-fifth (1.8%) normal saline with 4.3% glucose (dextrose saline) is an acceptable alternative to normal saline unless the patient has been taking copious drinks of water between vomiting attacks, thus diluting plasma chloride.

## 27.3  Acid-Base Balance

Readers should consult larger textbooks for the theoretical basis of acid-base balance in the body for it is a complex subject involving higher mathematical formulae. Disturbances of acid-base balance can be anticipated in the presence of respiratory or metabolic disorders, which can cause acidosis or alkalosis.

### 27.3.1  Respiratory Acidosis
Acidosis of respiratory origin arises when an increase in the blood carbon dioxide level and a fall in pH occurs in any of the following circumstances:

1) Obstruction of the upper respiratory tract by foreign bodies, tumours, inflammatory swellings or secretions

2) Trauma, e.g. multiple fractures of the ribs (stove-in chest) or open chest injury with pneumothorax

3) Chronic respiratory disease or pulmonary infections, interference with breathing after head injuries, or narcotic and barbiturate poisoning, meningitis and poliomyelitis

Respiratory acidosis is not accompanied by an electrolyte disturbance, and those with chronic respiratory insufficiency tolerate much higher blood carbon dioxide levels than normal subjects. The need for treatment depends on the distress or discomfort of the patient. Obstructive conditions require surgical removal of the obstruction or, if that is not possible, a tracheostomy.

It is particularly dangerous to administer respiratory depressant opiates to sufferers from chronic respiratory obstruction. Opiates reduce the sensitivity of the respiratory centres to carbon dioxide, reducing the effort to breathe and death from hypoxia can easily take place.

Acidosis of traumatic and medical origin can be relieved by mechanical ventilation and appropriate treatment of the cause of the condition. Such patients will tolerate light general anaesthesia and relaxants very satisfactorily.

### 27.3.2  Respiratory Alkalosis
Respiratory alkalosis is the result of over-breathing due to emotion, pain or stimulation of the respiratory centres by lesions of the central nervous system. Hyperventilation also occurs occasionally in liver failure. The symptoms include light-headedness and dizziness from depression of the arousal mechanism in the brain stem reticular formation. Increased muscular irritability (carpopedal spasm and a positive Chvostek's sign—

twitching of facial muscles following tapping on the facial nerve behind the ear) due to reduction of ionised calcium may also be present. The condition is no contra-indication to anaesthesia, but attention should be given to removing the cause and replacing calcium if signs of muscular irritability persist.

### 27.3.3 Metabolic Acidosis

Metabolic acidosis occurs from an accumulation of non-volatile acid in the bloodstream, with a reduction in plasma bicarbonate. It can arise from a variety of causes. Those encountered in anaesthesia include:

1) *Renal causes.* Patients with oliguria and vasoconstriction or urinary tract obstruction accumulate nitrogenous metabolites (urea, uric acid, creatinine). The body cannot excrete the hydrogen ions, which become attached to plasma bicarbonate with reduction of alkali reserve. Acidosis causes hyperventilation, which helps to eliminate some of the carbon dioxide and raise the blood pH, which may have fallen slightly.

2) *Oligaemia.* Acidosis due to oligaemia is reversible by intravenous therapy to restore renal activity, an essential measure before proceeding to surgery.

3) *Diabetes.* The presence of acidic ketone bodies in urine of diabetic patients causes acidosis and precedes the onset of coma. Correction is essential before surgery (see also Sect. 6.1).

4) *Hypoxia.* Any tissue becomes acidotic if deprived of oxygen. Respiratory failure and cardiac arrest are therefore high on the list of causal factors. Other causes are open-heart surgery, and replacement of the abdominal aorta. The possibility of hypoxia should be borne in mind when considering problems likely to arise in anaesthesia for these conditions.

5) *Ureterocolic transplantation.* Acidosis frequently occurs following transplant of the ureter into the colon. Urinary urea in the colon ferments and forms ammonia, which following reabsorption with chloride ions into the circulation results in a fall in plasma bicarbonate and a rise in plasma chloride.

Biochemical features of metabolic acidosis are a low blood pH and plasma bicarbonate, with a greatly increased $P\text{CO}_2$. The clinical features are those of the causal conditions, with drowsiness and some hyperventilation in addition.

Correction before anaesthesia is essential. If facilities for estimation of $P\text{CO}_2$ and pH are not available and clinical signs suggest acidosis, then slow infusion of 100 ml 8.4% sodium bicarbonate over 10 min is safe and will produce marked clinical improvement. If for any reason (anuria or congestive cardiac failure) the administration of sodium is contra-indicated, then intravenous THAM (trishydroxymethylaminomethane) solution 0.3 mol/l, at 5-10 ml/kg/h is worth a trial. This is a new agent but favourable reports have appeared following its use. Uraemic metabolic acidosis is an indication for haemodialysis.

### 27.3.4  Metabolic Alkalosis

There are various causes of metabolic alkalosis (excessive alkali therapy, diuretic therapy and loss of hydrogen ions) but of particular concern to anaesthetists are:

1) Loss of gastric secretions including hydrochloric acid from vomiting

2) Loss of potassium from intestinal fistulae

Drowsiness and fluid depletion require correction before anaesthesia. Treatment is aimed at restoring fluid depletion, with addition of potassium (potassium chloride, 25 mmol/l) to alternate litres of fluid replacement before anaesthesia. If calcium is deficient, 10 ml 10% calcium gluconate should also be added to the intravenous fluid used for replacement.

# 28 Some Common Emergency Procedures

28.1 Strangulated Hernia
28.2 Perforated Peptic Ulcer
28.3 Perforation of Large Intestine
28.4 Volvulus of Large Intestine
28.5 Haematemesis
28.6 Burst Abdomen

The hazards of orthopaedic and traumatic emergencies are discussed in Chap. 33 and those of vascular surgery in Chap 41. Among the commoner abdominal emergencies are strangulated hernia, intestinal obstruction, perforated peptic ulcer, perforation of the large intestine and diverticulitis, volvulus of the large intestine, haematemesis and burst abdomen.

## 28.1 Strangulated Hernia

If vomiting has been copious, patients are often dehydrated and require a drip and suction regime to correct fluid and electrolyte balance before surgery. Anaesthetic techniques popular for these conditions include low spinal or regional anaesthesia. Nausea associated with regional methods can be prevented by intravenous injection of 25 mg chlorpromazine and pethidine, after which patients sleep throughout the procedure.

## 28.2 Perforated Peptic Ulcer

Shock and dehydration may need correction. Stomach contents are a hazard but as often as not pass into the peritoneal cavity through the perforation. Intravenous infusion and maximal muscle relaxation are essential as vagotomy or partial gastrectomy is often undertaken. Risk of postoperative pulmonary complications is high and postoperative physiotherapy is advisable.

### 28.3  Perforation of Large Intestine

This carries a high mortality from endotoxin shock (see Sect. 26.3.3). Every effort must be made to reverse the vasoconstriction and restore good visceral perfusion before surgery, even if this means delay. Muscle relaxation is easily obtained as these patients have poorly developed abdominal muscles. Large doses are not necessary, especially if supplementary halothane is administered, thus avoiding difficulties sometimes encountered in the reversal of relaxant action.

### 28.4  Volvulus of Large Intestine

This is characterised by massive abdominal distension. Once the condition is relieved, uncomplicated recovery is usual.

### 28.5  Haematemesis

Prolonged blood transfusion after haematemesis often proves fruitless. Anaesthesia and surgery give better results if started early rather than late. Vigorous blood transfusion during surgery is essential until normal blood pressure returns and haemoglobin returns to 10-12 g/100 ml.

### 28.6  Burst Abdomen

Junior anaesthetists are often asked to anaesthetise for this condition. Patients are usually suffering from malnutrition, which is responsible for reduced powers of healing. Cardiovascular and respiratory state is often poor, with associated ileus and vomiting. Because of distension, maximum relaxation is essential to allow approximation of the wound. Repeated small doses of suxamethonium provide good operating conditions.

# Part IV

*Individual Types of Procedure*

# 29 Abdominal Surgery

## 29.1  Aim of Anaesthesia

The aim of anaesthesia for abdominal surgery is to produce maximum muscle relaxation with minimal physiological disturbance. In some circumstances this has been interpreted to mean minimal anaesthetic, on the assumption that anaesthetics produce more physiological disturbance than does surgical trauma. In the days before muscle relaxants, to secure acceptable muscle relaxation for upper abdominal surgery, anaesthesia with ether or chloroform almost to the point of respiratory arrest was necessary. It is not surprising therefore that there was a high incidence of postoperative cardiovascular and respiratory depression.

Since the introduction of relaxants, the pendulum has swung in the other direction. Some patients do not receive sufficient general anaesthetic to depress reflex autonomic responses to surgical trauma, which cause vasoconstriction, postoperative oxygen lack, poor urinary output and pulmonary complications. Too rapid return of consciousness and pain sensation, necessitating opiate sedation, contributes to cardiovascular instability. Inclusion of an inhalational agent or an intravenous opiate as part of the anaesthetic technique during abdominal operations makes sure that patients remain unconscious throughout and that recovery takes place gradually without restlessness.

## 29.2  Upper Abdominal Procedures

Operations on the gall bladder and bile ducts, the stomach, the spleen, the pancreas, the diaphragm and diaphragmatic hernias are usually referred to collectively as upper abdominal procedures.

A nasogastric tube should always be passed before or during any upper abdominal procedure. It should always be passed before induction in the presence of pyloric stenosis, gastric haemorrhage or obstruction. It is kinder to patients to wait until premedication has become effective. Passage after induction can conveniently be done with a well lubricated nasogastric tube placed inside a number 7 endotracheal tube which is passed blindly into the oesophagus through the nose. Sometimes direct vision with a laryngoscope is needed to direct the tube. The nasogastric tube is passed as far as possible into the abdomen before withdrawing the endotracheal tube. The catheter should be secured with a piece of tape in at least two places. Passage of the naso-endotracheal tube may cause temporary bleeding into the nose; the blood can be removed from the pharynx by suction.

### 29.2.1  Gall Bladder and Bile Ducts

Operations on the gall bladder and bile ducts require maximum relaxation.

When the common duct is opened, leakage of bile (especially if infected) may give rise to a period of vasoconstriction and shock during recovery which usually responds to oxygen therapy and intravenous fluids but can be significantly hastened by an intravenous injection of 10-25 mg chlorpromazine diluted in 10 ml saline.

### 29.2.2  Hiatus Hernia

Hiatus hernia also requires maximum relaxation, for the patients are often very fat and the surgeon is operating at the bottom of a deep hole.

### 29.2.3  Stomach

In gastric surgery full relaxation is necessary during manipulation and traction on mesenteries but is not necessary during the suturing of anastomoses. In rag and bottle days it was customary to lighten anaesthesia during suturing almost to the point of consciousness and deepen it again to allow closure of the peritoneum. Ventilation with a little halothane during the same phase lessens the total quantity of relaxants needed, whilst closure is often possible by adding a little halothane or thiopentone instead of further relaxant.

Total gastrectomy for malignant disease requires opening of the left side of the chest and removal of the spleen. The procedure is lengthy and blood loss usually underestimated.

Some anaesthetists pass a Robertshaw or Carlen tube to occlude the left main bronchus and allow total collapse of the left lung should the chest be opened. This is an anaesthetic refinement which inexperienced anaesthetists should avoid because satisfactory operating conditions can be provided with normal endotracheal anaesthesia. Indeed some surgeons prefer this method because it allows periodic inflation of areas of lung collapsed by pressure of retractors, etc.

Hiccup occurring when the duodenum is mobilised during gastrectomy has a nuisance value. It is not an indication for further muscle relaxant, which usually has no beneficial action. It arises from trauma to one of the crura of the diaphragm and is spasmodic. It is rarely seen in patients who have received intravenous chlorpromazine or who are under ether anaesthesia. When it occurs the best course is to increase the concentration of the inhalational agent chosen for the procedure. Addition of a muscle relaxant is ineffective.

Patients undergoing selective vagotomy are often denied premedication with atropine or halothane anaesthesia because it is thought that these drugs interfere with tests for the presence or absence of vagal activity. Absence of atropine is associated with excessive sweating and salivation. Electrical stimulation for vagal activity is not affected by premedication with pethidine and promethazine, or by halothane.

### 29.2.4  Spleen

Splenectomy is usually performed for blood dyscrasia or Banti's disease. The organ is large and fibrotic and sudden haemorrhage may occur from torn veins, especially the gastrosplenic groups or the splenic vein itself. A free-running intravenous line should be established before surgery begins.

### 29.2.5  Liver Disease

Sufferers from cirrhosis of the liver develop portal hypertension. Operations such as portacaval anastomosis, splenorenal anastomosis and proximal gastric transection involving ligation of vascular connections between stomach and oesophagus are often undertaken. The hazards of such procedures include operative haemorrhage, interference with blood clotting and reduced tolerance to opiates. Liver function is always depressed and if serum albumin is less than 3.2% the operation should not proceed.

Intravenous agents should be used with caution and pre-operative opiates avoided altogether. Even a small amount of pethidine (25-50 mg) can put a patient who is on the brink of liver failure into a state of coma.

During anaesthesia the main reliance should be placed on inhalational agents and non-depolarising relaxants. Inhalational agents can be eliminated through the lungs and do not require metabolism, and the action of non-depolarising relaxants can be reversed with neostigmine and atropine. A low serum cholinesterase level contra-indicates the use of suxamethonium and shortens the action of non-depolarising agents.

### 29.2.6 Oesophagus

Oesophagectomy is usually undertaken for malignant disease and is a lengthy procedure involving the abdominal cavity as well as the thorax. Depending on the site of the constriction, the aim of the operation is to restore continuity either by transposition of the large bowel to make a false oesophagus, if the constriction is high, or by anastomosis to the jejunum, if the constriction is at a lower level.

Careful assessment of patients is necessary since malnutrition and anaemia as well as electrolyte disturbances may require correction before operation and this may take several days.

The operation itself is lengthy, involves opening the thorax and can be associated with considerable blood loss, whilst the extensive tissue disturbance gives rise to postoperative shock.

Most anaesthetists base their technique on thiopentone relaxant and light general anaesthetic with nitrous oxide, oxygen and a little halothane, and keep shock to a minimum by accurate replacement of lost blood. The author prefers to include chlorpromazine in the premedication and in the anaesthetic technique with the object of reducing the incidence of postoperative shock and fluid retention.

After the operation, expert chest physiotherapy is vital (if necessary under light general anaesthesia or intravenous analgesia), to ensure expansion and aeration of the lung in the left chest.

### 29.2.7 Postoperative Pulmonary Complications

Pulmonary complications are more frequent after upper abdominal surgery than after lower abdominal surgery and this is partly the result of restricted breathing from the pain of the wound. Generous pain relief (20 mg papaveretum 4-hourly for 48 h) and deep breathing under supervision of a physiotherapist are routine preventive measures. Entonox inhalation has been used to reduce the pain of postoperative chest physiotherapy.

## 29.3  Lower Abdominal Procedures

Gynaecological and urological procedures are dealt with separately in Chaps. 30 and 32. Major procedures in the lower abdomen include hemicolectomy and anterior resection (sigmoid colectomy) for malignant disease or for Crohn's disease, total colectomy with ileorectal anastomosis or ileostomy for ulcerative colitis, and abdominoperineal excision for malignant disease of the rectum.

### 29.3.1  Hemicolectomy

Hemicolectomy for malignant disease presents no particular hazard. Patients with Crohn's disease, however, have usually been treated with steroids and will need cover during surgery (see Sect. 7.1). Total colectomy for ulcerative colitis is a less severe procedure than might be expected, provided that steroid cover is adequate. If the rectum is excised as well, haemorrhage is brisk and postoperative oozing will be considerable.

### 29.3.2  Excision of Rectum

Abdominoperineal excision of the rectum for malignant disease is more extensive and includes excision of the inferior mesenteric lymph nodes and wide pelvic removal. Two surgeons usually operate, one on the abdomen and one on the perineum, in what is called the synchronous combined excision.

Positioning of patient and instruments for two surgical teams takes about half an hour. Anaesthetists should ensure the security of their intravenous infusion and monitoring equipment, because access during the procedure with so many people around is virtually impossible. Patients are usually put in the lithotomy position with a modest head-down tilt. The perineal area is quite invisible to the anaesthetist who should ask to be informed when the perineal operation begins, because of the accompanying haemorrhage. It is surprising how often surgical or nursing teams fail to do this.

An alternative method used by surgeons who like to do all their own operating is to complete the first part and the colostomy and close the abdomen with the patient supine and in a modest Trendelenburg position, and then to turn the patient into the lateral position for completion of the perineal part of the operation. Movement at this stage is inconvenient to the anaesthetist and particular care is needed to preserve the integrity of intravenous infusion and the connections between the patient and the apparatus. If subdural or epidural analgesia is being used, some fall in blood pressure may take place, but this can be offset by maintaining the modest head-down tilt.

Some degree of controlled hypotension can reduce blood loss during the perineal stage, whilst long acting spinal analgesia with light general anaesthetic cover has been deservedly popular in the past.

Postoperative oozing from the perineum often exceeds 1 litre during 24 h, and allowance should be made for this when arranging blood replacement.

Some surgeons place antibiotics in the peritoneal cavity after surgery of the colon, of which some (e.g. erythromycin) prolong the action of muscle relaxants. Intestinal movement after reversal of non-depolarising relaxants with neostigmine and atropine was at one time thought to prejudice the security of colonic anastomoses. These fears have not been substantiated.

### 29.3.3   Herniorrhaphy

Adequate relaxation for the average inguinal or femoral hernia can be obtained with 2% halothane. Intubation is optional.

Large sliding and umbilical hernias containing omentum and bowel require full relaxation, intubation and intravenous therapy. Large umbilical hernias are prevalent in very fat women with chronic bronchitis and high blood pressure. If the hernias contain bowel, multiple adhesions will require separation and blood loss may be considerable; therefore blood should be cross-matched beforehand. If blood is not available, fresh frozen plasma or dextran 70 should be administered.

After operation sometimes inadequate respiration will require treatment on a ventilator. Indications are discussed in Chap. 24.

### 29.3.4   Diverticulitis and Pelvic Abscesses

Laparotomy for diverticulitis carries a strong risk of endotoxic shock following excision of inflamed bowel, drainage of a pelvic abscess or peritonitis following perforation. The latter is usually of great severity and has high mortality.

When it is necessary to undertake surgical drainage of the peritoneum or of pelvic abscesses, consideration should be given to doing these under cover of cortisone or chlorpromazine. In both, protective action against endotoxin exceeds their curative effect. This is fully discussed in Chap. 26.

# 30 Gynaecological Surgery

The hazards of anaesthesia for gynaecological surgery do not differ materially from those for abdominal surgery. There are, however, exceptions, as a brief review of gynaecological procedures will reveal.

## 30.1 Vaginal Procedures

Vaginal procedures include plastic repair for prolapse of bladder and rectum (sometimes together with vaginal hysterectomy); dilatation and curettage; termination of pregnancy; insufflation of fallopian tubes for treatment of infertility or severance for sterilization.

### 30.1.1 Plastic Repair

Plastic repair procedures include repair of prolapse, amputation of the cervix, and vaginal hysterectomy. Haemorrhage may be brisk but usually not prolonged, so an intravenous infusion is optional. Blood loss can be reduced by epidural or spinal techniques (Chap. 17), controlled hypotension (Chap. 19), or local infiltration with normal saline containing 1:200 000 adrenaline.

Although adrenaline, when associated with halothane anaesthesia, is theoretically a cardiovascular hazard, dilute solutions appear to be harmless, provided both the anaesthetist and surgeon check the strength of adrenaline before addition to the saline solution. Nevertheless anaesthetists should discourage a practice of questionable benefit and possible harm (see also Sect. 12.5.4).

### 30.1.2 Dilatation and Curettage

Dilatation for diagnostic purposes, the cervix being closed, requires a reasonable depth of anaesthesia to avoid laryngospasm and cardiac irregularity.

If the purpose is curettage for miscarriage, the cervix is usually partially opened and light anaesthesia is adequate. The range of suitable anaesthetic agents is wide and endotracheal intubation unnecessary. Maintenance of a clear airway for such a short procedure should be within the competence even of beginners, and offers valuable training experience.

### 30.1.3   Termination of Pregnancy

Uterine haemorrhage constitutes a special hazard of termination of pregnancy, for which reason halothane, with its property of relaxing smooth muscle, is an unpopular agent, although if it is given in a low concentration the liability to postoperative haemorrhage is not increased. Nevertheless, if the surgeon expresses dislike for the agent, plenty of alternatives are available, e.g. trichloroethylene, methoxyflurane, or intravenous techniques. Intravenous injection of ergotamine, when the uterus has been emptied, stimulates uterine contraction. A theoretical hazard exists, since ergotamine increases venous and arterial tone, possibly causing angina or acute pulmonary oedema in patients with pre-existing heart disease. The author has used this agent for many years and never seen such adverse reactions, possibly because advanced heart disease is rare in women of child-bearing age.

## 30.2   Abdominal Pelvic Operations

The commoner elective abdominal pelvic operations include ovariectomy, salpingo-oophorectomy, broad ligament cysts, endometriosis, hyster-ectomy for fibroids or neoplasms, and occasionally, pelvic clearance for advanced malignant conditions. All these operations are carried out with a head-down tilt (Trendelenburg position), the hazards of which have been discussed in Chap. 15. This position does not cause respiratory embarrassment in the average patient, but may do so in those who are obese.

Ovarian cysts vary in size. Large cysts can occupy the entire abdomen, causing respiratory embarrassment. Intubation is advisable, but only a short-acting relaxant is necessary, since no further relaxation is needed after the abdomen is opened, as the muscles are already stretched. In spite of the size of the tumours, these operations are usually completed without any particular complication.

Malignant ovarian cysts are often accompanied by ascites. If it causes embarrassment to breathing, the fluid should be aspirated before induction of anaesthesia, but patients should be spared such an unpleasant procedure if possible.

Broad ligament cysts, endometriosis ('chocolate cysts') and salpingo-oophorectomy take time but are not usually accompanied by much haemorrhage. Hysterectomy for small tumours is a relatively simple operation, but when fibroids are large, access to the main blood vessels around the cervix becomes difficult and sudden haemorrhage can occur. Wertheim's total hysterectomy and pelvic clearance carry the same hazards as other extensive procedures, namely haemorrhage and operative shock. Adequate supplies of cross-matched blood are essential and techniques to reduce bleeding, e.g. spinal, epidural, or controlled hypotension are helpful for surgeons and beneficial to patients.

Anaesthetic techniques for all these operation are straightforward, and thiopentone, relaxant, intubation and maintenance with nitrous oxide, oxygen and halothane is probably the commonest, except as mentioned for the radical operations.

Since relaxation for pelvic surgery is relatively easy to obtain, satisfactory operating conditions can easily be provided by inhalational agents and spontaneous respiration without need for intubation, as patients are already in the head-down position.


## 30.3  Laparoscopy

The hazards of anaesthesia for laparoscopy have been much underrated. Inadequate control of the volume of gas entering the abdominal cavity has obstructed diaphragmatic movement, with cardiorespiratory embarrassment sufficient to cause cardiac arrest. Passage of gases through defects in the diaphragm has resulted in pneumothorax, and if on the left side, cardiac tamponade. Injection of carbon dioxide can increase the plasma carbon dioxide and blood pressure as well as causing cardiac irregularities. Perforation of the bowel and regurgitation and pulmonary aspiration of stomach content after failure to intubate have also been reported.

The potential dangers of laparoscopy are now more generally appreciated, following publication of reports about mishaps. Preventive measures include measurement of pressures and volumes of injected gases: the intra-abdominal pressure is not allowed to exceed 4 kPa. Nitrous oxide has replaced carbon dioxide, eliminating the side-effects of that agent. Anaesthesia for laparoscopy should not be assigned to unsupervised trainees. Endotracheal intubation with controlled respiration is usual with continuous monitoring of pulse and blood pressure particularly during insufflation. Lighting should not be lowered to facilitate viewing through the laparoscope until the insufflation is completed and it is clear that no ill effects have resulted. Even so, an independent source of illumination is needed for anaesthetists to check the gas flows, the presence or absence of cyanosis or deficient capillary perfusion.

## 30.4   Ruptured Ectopic Gestation

Rupture of a tubal pregnancy can be accompanied by a catastrophic haemorrhage. Patients often appear to be 'bled white' and become moribund with imperceptible pulse and unrecordable blood pressure. Vein constriction may be so intense as to require a 'cut-down' or use of a femoral or jugular vein to establish an intravenous line. In spite of such discouraging appearances, anaesthesia should never be withheld, however hopeless the case may seem. As soon as an intravenous infusion is started with fresh frozen plasma or dextran and recordable blood pressure obtained, anaesthesia can begin. All intravenous agents should be avoided, induction being with pure oxygen and an inhalational agent, either ether or halothane. As soon as the conjunctival reflexes have vanished (first plane, third stage) the operation may begin; prostration is so extreme that muscle relaxants are not necessary. As soon as the abdomen is opened and blood clots removed from the peritoneum, the patient's condition improves and the pulse becomes palpable.

The author has confirmed this observation in the past under conditions when intravenous methods were not available. Removal of the blood clot reduces the reflex sympathetic constriction evoked by its presence and previously absent temporal pulsation reappears. Relaxing of the arterioles lowers vasomotor tone or critical closing pressure (see Chap. 20), with improved peripheral perfusion.

# 31 Operative Obstetrics

The hazards of obstetric anaesthesia are unique in that they concern two persons, the unborn child and the mother. The hazards for the unborn child are a reflection of the anaesthetic techniques employed, which in recent years have tended to confer marginal benefits to the child at what some may consider an unjustifiable cost to the mother in terms of awareness during delivery.

## 31.1  Passage of Drugs Across the Placenta

Apart from the dangers to the child of oxygen lack during anaesthesia—dangers usually shared by the mother, but also a possible result of excessive uterine contraction—respiratory depression in the neonate immediately after delivery can arise from transmission of anaesthetics, sedative drugs and muscle relaxants across the placenta.

Any substance in maternal blood can cross the placental barrier to some extent, unless altered or destroyed during passage. Drugs with high lipoid solubility, including general anaesthetics, and drugs with low molecular weight (up to 600) cross the placenta rapidly, non-ionised ones crossing more rapidly than ionised. All general anaesthetics cross the placenta.

### 31.1.1  General Anaesthetics
Opinions differ about the extent to which thiopentone enters the fetal

circulation. It is generally taught that the placenta offers no barrier to thiopentone and that maximum fetal blood levels coincide with the onset of maternal anaesthesia, subsequently falling slowly. Hence fetal depression would be at a maximum soon after induction, but considerably less if a delay of 5-7 min took place.

More recent animal experimentation using radioactive thiopentone has shown delay in passage across the placenta, so that fetal blood levels are less than those of the mother at the onset of anaesthesia.

Experience suggests this may also be true in humans, since fetal respiratory depression was not a prominent feature when induction with 500 mg thiopentone was withheld until skin preparation and towelling were completed; rapid delivery followed. For many years this was routine in the author's practice.

All inhalational agents pass the placental barrier. Over many years in practice, however, respiratory depression of infants was by no means consistently related to the particular agent used, whether ether, cyclo-propane, trichloroethylene, or halothane.

Opiates pass the placental barrier, and depress respiration of the new-born child, but pethidine less than morphine. Nevertheless, administration should be avoided within 3 h of delivery (admittedly very difficult to predict).

The respiratory depressant effect of opiates can be reversed, in the child or in the mother, by the use of morphine antagonists: nalorphine or naloxone. For a new-born baby, an appropriate dose can be injected into the umbilical vein and repeated if necessary. Morphine or opiate antagonists, besides reversing respiratory depression, also decrease their analgesic effects.

The tranquillising phenothiazines chlorpromazine, promethazine and promazine also cross the placental barrier, but do not depress fetal respiration. When administered together with pethidine, they reduce the respiratory depressant effect by 50%. Their anti-emetic and tranquillising action is also of immense benefit to an anxious primipara, preventing nausea and vomiting, on which pethidine has no effect.

Hyoscine hydrobromide has an amnesic action and little adverse effect on the unborn child. Given late during childbirth, however, it may cause restlessness and disorientation of the mother.

### 31.1.2  Relaxants

In large doses, relaxants can cross the placental barrier in sufficient quantities to affect the fetus, but clinical doses are without harmful effect, although most anaesthetists avoid gallamine in obstetrics, since it is reputed to cross more rapidly than other relaxants.

### 31.1.3  Local Analgesics

Whether used for epidural, caudal, paracervical or pudendal blocks, all local analgesics rapidly find their way into the fetal circulation but seldom cause disturbance.

Sometimes after attempted paracervical block, absorption of the local analgesic is particularly rapid, owing to the dilatation of the blood vessels, and adverse effects on the fetus show themselves by bradycardia and increase in movements, indicating need to accelerate delivery.

## 31.2 Hazards to the Mother

The major hazard to the mother in obstetrical anaesthesia is lack of experience of anaesthetists, particularly when they attempt to carry out unfamiliar techniques.

Inhalation of regurgitated gastric contents, resulting in asphyxia by obstruction or fatal pneumonitis (Mendelson's syndrome) is one cause of anaesthetic maternal death. Another is cardiac arrest before, during or after delivery, from respiratory obstruction and oxygen lack. Failed or difficult intubation accounts for at least 25% of deaths in this category. Other causes include respiratory obstruction during induction or during the operative procedure itself, unrecognised because the anaesthetist's attention has been diverted by other problems, such as the condition of the new-born child or attention to intravenous drips.

A less common hazard is severe drop in blood pressure due to the gravid uterus pressing on the inferior vena cava when the patient is in the supine position. This complication can demonstrate itself in an alarming fashion following relaxation of the abdominal muscles by regional (epidural or subdural) techniques or the action of muscle relaxants. The gravid uterus, no longer supported by muscle tone in the abdomen, falls back on the inferior vena cava and interferes with the return of blood from the lower extremities. Hypotension from this cause can be avoided by adopting a left lateral tilt as a routine before and after local blocks or before induction of general anaesthesia. A left tilt will always restore stability of circulation.

Recovery is not without its hazards. Cardiac arrest has been described from untreated respiratory depression by opiates, from unreversed muscular paralysis and from respiratory obstruction. Detection of cyanosis is difficult and uncertain in dark-skinned patients, especially when illumination is by blue-tinted strip-lighting (see Sect. 22.2). Recovery facilities in isolated obstetric units and small maternity hospitals are often inadequate. Even in general hospitals with a small emergency turnover, recovery rooms are often closed at night—precisely when they may most be needed for obstetric patients. It should be a rule in all obstetric units that anaesthetists never leave an unconscious patient until satisfied that the airway is clear, that breathing is adequate and that a nurse experienced in recovery is in charge.

### 31.3   Preventing Aspiration of Gastric Contents

*31.3.1   Equipment*

No obstetric anaesthetic should be undertaken without suitable equipment for dealing with regurgitation of stomach contents, and the presence of an experienced assistant. Minimal equipment requirements include:

1) A tipping table

2) Efficient suction and sucker ends (metal is easier to handle than plastic)

3) Two laryngoscopes, assorted endotracheal tubes and connections

4) *Transparent* face masks

5) A modern anaesthetic apparatus

6) Bronchoscopes and bronchoscopic suckers

7) Anaesthetic agents, muscle relaxants and emergency drugs, including atropine, ergotamine, respiratory stimulants and opiate antagonists

Careful attention should be devoted to storage and maintenance of equipment. Too often the items are stored in different cupboards and valuable time is wasted in their collection and assembly. In smaller units the apparatus may occupy a corner of the delivery room, covered with towels, and go unchecked between one anaesthetic and another.

A qualified specialist (a consultant anaesthetist) should be in charge of anaesthetic arrangements in an obstetric unit (in Great Britain this is now accepted policy), and one of the consultant's duties should be to ensure that all anaesthetic and ancillary equipment, drugs, etc. are ready for use at a moment's notice and are checked every day.

*31.3.2   Patient Care*

Prevention of the hazard of regurgitation of stomach contents begins with the admission of the patient to the obstetric department. Once childbirth has started, a regime should be instituted to keep stomach contents to a minimum and ensure reduction of acidity to a pH of 12.5 or above. Recent research suggests that it is not the pH of the fluid, but the mere presence of water which has an adverse effect on the pulmonary epithelium. Reports of two fatalities from aspiration of alkalinised stomach content would appear to confirm this suggestion. Nevertheless the policy of keeping stomach contents alkaline must be strictly observed. Patients can be divided into *'low-risk'* and *'high-risk'* classes.

*Low-risk* patients are those who are not expected to require a general anaesthetic. They are allowed a light, easily digestible diet during childbirth, avoiding fats, milk, etc. Sieved foods are suitable and drinks should not contain more than 5% glucose, for strengths above this delay emptying time. All receive 15 ml magnesium trisilicate or aluminium hydroxide every 2 h until delivery. Since pain, sedatives and emotion all contribute to delay in the emptying time of the stomach, a tablet of metoclopramide should be taken after each feed to speed up emptying time.

*High-risk* patients include those whose previous obstetric history suggests that an anaesthetic may be needed for delivery or who have disproportion, multiple pregnancies or malposition of the fetus. They should receive *nothing* by mouth. An intravenous drip of 5% glucose, 1 litre every 2 h, supplies fluid and calories from the onset of childbirth. In addition the patients receive the routine alkaline oral medication already described.

### 31.3.3  Local Analgesia

Since aspiration of stomach contents remains a major cause of maternal mortality in obstetrical anaesthesia, it is very logical to make use of regional methods (subdural, epidural, pudendal blocks, etc.) whenever possible.

Epidural analgesia is gaining popularity, and where staff are available it is offered to all patients in childbirth, irrespective of whether operative interference is likely or not, as well as to those requiring caesarean section. The hazards of this particular procedure are dealt with in Sect. 17.3.

The main hazard of epidural technique is inadvertent overdose. In the last confidential survey in Great Britain, there were two anaesthetic deaths attributable to epidural methods. One of these was from an inadvertent but massive overdose. This is not quoted to discourage the use of the method, but only as a warning once more of the need for experience in whatever method is used.

Subdural (spinal analgesia) has advocates especially in the United States, where low spinal ('saddle' block) is widely used for operative vaginal deliveries. In one series over 15 000 patients were treated in this way without a fatality. The method is also very suitable for caesarean section.

Whatever the technique (epidural or subdural) an intravenous infusion is essential and should initially run at a fast rate to compensate for the increase in vascular capacity accompanying sympathetic blockade.

A *left lateral tilt* should be adopted in all patients to avoid hypotension from the pressure of the gravid uterus on the inferior vena cava when using epidural or spinal techniques. (Failure in the past to recognise this syndrome and to take appropriate avoiding action is one reason why spinal analgesia is not more widely used in obstetrics.)

### 31.3.4  General Anaesthesia

Having ensured that, as far as possible, the patient's stomach contains no food and has alkaline contents, general anaesthetic techniques are directed at prevention of vomiting during induction and recovery, and at prevention of regurgitation once unconsciousness has been produced.

When gastric contents are known or suspected to exist, for example in emergency, a number 10 nasogastric tube should be passed to aspirate any contents present. It is quite likely that the patient will vomit during the procedure and empty the stomach herself. Intravenous apomorphine in a dose of 3 mg to induce nausea has also been advocated, but those with experience of this procedure consider it too unpleasant to be justified.

Current teaching on avoiding regurgitation of stomach contents during obstetric anaesthesia has become so dogmatic that many anaesthetists honestly believe the only safe way of achieving this end is by 'crash' induction. There is, however, a growing appreciation that alternatives exist that are equally safe for the mother and less exacting for the anaesthetist, but which possibly expose the unborn child to a marginal degree of respiratory depression. The choice depends mainly on the experience and skill of the operator. Methods familiar to one anaesthetist may be beyond the capacity of another, who will achieve better results by simpler methods.

There are three methods in current use:

1) Crash induction: intravenous induction, quick-acting relaxant, intubation and maintenance with nitrous oxide and oxygen

2) Rapid intravenous induction, paralysis with a longer-acting relaxant, maintenance with nitrous oxide, oxygen and 0.5% halothane

3) Induction of anaesthesia in the lateral position with inhalational agents only and subsequent intubation at the discretion of the anaesthetist

*Crash Induction.* The widely taught method of crash induction involves atropine 0.5 mg premedication, 3 min preoxygenation with the patient in the steep head-up position, followed by induction of anaesthesia with up to 250 mg of 2.5% thiopentone, followed immediately by 50-100 mg intravenous suxamethonium. At this point, an assistant applies cricoid pressure, whilst the anaesthetist passes and inflates a cuffed endotracheal tube. From then on, anaesthesia is maintained with 30% oxygen and 70% nitrous oxide with supplementary relaxants as needed until the child is delivered, after which anaesthesia can be continued with additional inhalational agents of choice, or small doses of intravenous opiate.

This method provides optimum conditions for the unborn child, but can require a high degree of expertise in endotracheal intubation, as well as the knowledge that on occasion direct intubation may not be possible and recourse may have to be had to other means of anaesthesia.

The weakness of crash induction lies in the fact that in the interval between the action of suxamethonium and the passage of the tube, the trachea and bronchial tree are virtually unprotected against the entrance of any fluid or foreign matter, which can easily occur after administration of suxamethonium.

The muscle fasciculations accompanying the action of suxamethonium can cause a brief but substantial rise in intra-abdominal pressure, from the normal 1.0-1.2 kPa to exceed 1.9 kPa in 12% of patients. Should the stomach contain any fluid, this brief rise in pressure is sufficient (in accordance with the law of Laplace) to open the cardio-oesophageal junction, and project stomach content into the pharynx from whence oxygen insufflation can drive it into the lungs.

To overcome this, steep foot-down tilt has been recommended. Intragastric pressure at term is 1.0-1.2 kPa and regurgitation of stomach contents does not occur until intragastric pressure reaches 1.8 kPa. In order to raise the larynx the necessary 19 cm above the cardio-oesophageal junction, a foot-down tilt of 40° is required. In this position, should regurgitation occur, there would be no time (even with a specially equipped table) to reverse to a 15°-20° head-down tilt before fluid entered the trachea and bronchi.

A foot-down tilt being no guarantee against regurgitation, it is better to avoid the method and employ Sellick's manoeuvre of cricoid compression instead. The only disadvantage of this procedure is that displacement of the larynx can add to intubation problems (see below).

The second hazard of a crash induction is the short time available for intubation before the action of suxamethonium wears off. Women of childbearing age usually have a full dentition, which increases difficulties in visualisation of the larynx (see Sect. 14.2). Furthermore, at full term, water retention increases the size of the tongue. In some units patients are anaesthetised for operative obstetrics on their bed, which also adds to difficulties of intubation.

Finally, if the obstetrician and assistants are waiting scrubbed-up, an atmosphere of impatience may lead anaesthetists to rush their fences and create more intubation problems than would occur in a calmer atmosphere.

Sometimes, if the first attempts to intubate are unsuccessful, following insufflation with oxygen, a further attempt is made just as laryngeal reflexes begin to return, resulting in laryngeal spasm accompanied by expulsive efforts which can increase intragastric pressure sufficiently to open the cardio-oesophageal junction and project stomach content into the pharynx. After a further dose of suxamethonium has restored tranquillity, cyanosis will require insufflation with oxygen prior to resumption of attempts to intubate. At this time any stomach content in the pharynx is driven directly through an unprotected larynx into the trachea and bronchi, all expulsive effort being impossible.

Experienced anaesthetists can avoid this contretemps by (a) anticipating the need for further relaxant and avoiding spasm, or (b) suction of the pharynx before insufflation, should spasm have occurred. Less experienced anaesthetists in the stress of the moment often neglect to do either.

*Modified Crash Induction.* For junior anaesthetists and those who find crash induction too stressful, an alternative, modified crash induction consists of intravenous induction as for a crash induction, but administration of a longer-acting and more gradually reversed relaxant. The recently introduced fazadinium has a rapid action and lasts 15-20 min, and it appears very suitable. Alcuronium has had its advocates, and pancuronium is equally effective but takes longer to act. These agents give ample time to overcome any difficulties in intubation whilst avoiding muscle spasm and increase in intragastric pressure.

Failure to intubate is an acknowledged hazard of crash induction. Attempts at intubation should be limited and an alternative routine in case of failure agreed beforehand.

It has been stated that silent regurgitation and aspiration of stomach contents can occur in a spontaneously breathing and surgically anaesthetised patient. This is contrary to the experience of anaesthetists who began their anaesthetic career before the introduction of muscle relaxants; they would agree that, in normal patients, if the vomiting reflex is suppressed, no material can regurgitate from the stomach into the oesophagus, no matter what position the patient is in so long as the cardio-oesophageal valve sphincter mechanism is not interfered with.

Regurgitation and aspiration of stomach contents were unknown when old-fashioned rag and bottle methods were used for obstetrical anaesthesia. Figures produced for the Birmingham area in 1954 revealed that no mortality or morbidity of any significance accompanied anaesthesia for domiciliary midwifery, where rag and bottle methods were the rule. These findings received support from other parts of the country. Experience in a large maternity hospital in Singapore for the 11 years preceding the introduction of relaxants or thiopentone, showed that open-drop ether given by junior residents was perfectly safe and not accompanied by inhalation of gastric contents. When thiopentone was introduced for obstetrical anaesthesia, two deaths occurred in 6 months.

Mendelson's syndrome arose from inexperience and resulted from the severe laryngospasm accompanied by unrecognised regurgitation of stomach contents during anaesthesia induced with nitrous oxide, oxygen and ether, a difficult technique needing skill and experience. Mendelson himself (who was not an anaesthetist) laid the blame on:

1) Assignation of 'new and inexperienced' interns to obstetrics work

2) Rushing an active patient into the delivery room and inducing general anaesthesia with an opaque mask fastened by harness on the face

3) Failure of an anaesthetist to observe the presence of cyanosis, or of the vomit and gastric contents which the opaque mask so often conceals

*General Anaesthesia Without Intubation.* Failure to intubate or lack of knowledge of how to intubate means that the patients will have to receive an inhalational anaesthesia. The hazards of this procedure are admittedly those of vomiting and regurgitation as for any other anaesthetic.

Before induction a number 10 nasogastric tube should be passed for aspiration of any stomach contents.

Induction should be by inhalational methods only, intravenous induction being unsuitable because of the possibility of increased intra-gastric pressure from coughing and spasm. For induction the patient should be in the left lateral position with the head low. Any vomiting will occur before loss of consciousness, laryngeal and cough reflexes remaining active and respiration being inhibited during the expulsive act of vomiting. In the lateral position, gravity assisted by suction ensures that stomach contents flow out of the mouth onto the pillow. Consciousness rapidly returns to allow clearance of the pharynx by coughing and spitting, after which induction can be resumed. Vomiting during induction was rare with open-drop chloroform, which may explain its former popularity.

Once the patient is anaesthetised, regurgitation is unlikely, unless there is excessive pressure on the upper abdomen. Vaginal delivery can take place in the lateral position, but if caesarean section is necessary, the patient can be turned into the supine position with a modest head-down and left lateral tilt and the operation proceed.

The choice of inhalational agent depends on whether any method of analgesia has been used in the hours preceding the induction of general anaesthesia. If trichloroethylene or methoxyflurane has been admin-istered to produce analgesia, it is logical to continue the use of the same agent to produce full anaesthesia, as the blood content is already somewhat raised. If the patient has received no general anaesthetic, halothane with oxygen would appear to be the agent of choice. It has been credited with the following desirable properties for obstetrical anaesthesia:

1) Induction is rapid.
2) Relaxation is soon obtained.
3) Laryngospasm does not occur.
4) Secretions, salivary or bronchial, are slight.
5) Vomiting during induction or recovery is rare.
6) Recovery is rapid.

Two disadvantages are its hypotensive effect and relaxation of uterine muscle, fully discussed in Chap. 12.

The hypotensive and muscle relaxant properties of chloroform are far greater than those of halothane, and in addition it is an acknowledged liver poison. In spite of these properties many obstetricians preferred it to ether and other agents for almost 100 years.

*Ketamine.* Patients under the influence of ketamine retain their swallowing reflexes, a useful property in obstetrical anaesthesia. Ketamine has provided satisfactory anaesthesia for forceps deliveries and for induction before caesarean section, and there is no reason why (in the absence of skilled anaesthetists) it should not be employed for the entire procedure.

The progress of investigations into its use in obstetrics was halted when radio-opaque substances placed in the pharynx were shown to enter the trachea and bronchi during anaesthesia with ketamine. Subsequent investigations have failed to confirm this finding. In clinical doses the laryngeal reflexes remain fully active. Since the radio-opaque substances used are non-irritant (and used in any case for bronchograms) one would expect them to pass the larynx without much response, in contrast to more irritant substances.

Eclampsia is a contra-indication to the use of ketamine, because its sympathetic stimulatory properties can increase systolic blood pressure.


## 31.4 Summary

Hazards of obstetrical anaesthesia can best be avoided by:

1) Appointing experienced anaesthetists to organise and administer obstetrical anaesthetic services and train junior anaesthetists, nursing and technical staff

2) Teaching techniques suitable to the experience and skills of those expected to carry them out

3) Anaesthetic obstetrical training that includes a statutory period of 3 months whole-time residence in an obstetric unit of 40 beds or more, the trainee attending *in person* all deliveries, whether they are carried out under regional or general anaesthesia, as well as supervising administration of analgesia during childbirth

# 32 Urological Surgery

Urological procedures include operations on the kidney, ureter, bladder, prostate gland and urethra, operations for phaeochromocytoma, sex-change procedures, and renal transplantation.

## 32.1 Kidney

*32.1.1 Approaches*
The kidney is usually approached either through the loin, with the patient in the lateral position, or transabdominally, with the patient supine. The disadvantages of the lateral position are set out in Sect. 15.5. Because the lateral position interferes with respiration and because the pleura may be opened during removal of a rib to improve access, endotracheal intubation, full relaxation and controlled respiration are essential, although only moderate muscular relaxation is required.

Aids to expose the kidney and bring it up into the wound include breaking the table, using the kidney bridge, and placing an inflatable cushion under the dependent loin. All have an adverse effect on the circulation, as they interfere with venous return through the inferior vena cava, which may even become kinked. The inflatable cushion causes least disturbance. Pulse and blood pressure should be kept under constant

review for at least 5 min after the manoeuvre has been carried out, and
the surgeon should be informed of any cardiovascular changes which the
anaesthetist finds unacceptable. Cardiovascular changes may be even
more marked in patients who have been completely relaxed with spinal or
epidural analgesia.

The transabdominal approach is less often used. It has obvious
advantages in extensive removal of kidney and ureter for neoplastic
conditions, as well as for examination of both kidneys.

### 32.1.2  Haemorrhage

Haemorrhage during operations on the kidney is not usually severe and
even during partial resection is usually well controlled. During the actual
removal of a kidney if a clamp on the renal pedicle slips, haemorrhage
from the renal vein or artery can be catastrophic. Rapid infusion (by a
pump) with the patient in the head-down position is the best treatment
until the surgeon regains control over the blood vessels.

### 31.1.3  Grawitz's Tumour

Carcinoma of the kidney is a highly vascular tumour. Haemorrhage may
be severe during its removal. The tumour sometimes extends along the
renal vein to the inferior vena cava. Small emboli may become detached
during the operation and cause cardiac arrest or delayed return of
consciousness, paraplegia or respiratory failure. Preventive action is
quite impossible. If the central nervous system is affected, 1 g hydrocortisone given intravenously may reduce cerebral oedema.

## 32.2  Renal Transplantation

Renal transplantation has hazards for donors and anaesthetists as well as
for patients.

### 32.2.1  Donor

Donors of kidneys are either relatives of acceptable tissue type, identical
twins or moribund victims of irreversible cerebral damage.

Related donors undergo nephrectomy at the same time as the recipient
is being made ready to receive the kidney. The rather tense and dramatic
atmosphere surrounding the recipient can indirectly have an adverse
effect on the donor, insofar as the conduct of anaesthesia may be left to a
junior, the senior electing to care for the recipient. Such an arrangement
may explain reports of healthy donors dying under anaesthesia. Kidney
recipients live on borrowed time. Healthy donors, although reducing
their life expectancy by giving away a kidney, can reasonably expect to
attain a ripe old age and should receive the highest anaesthetic skills
available, always at consultant level.

Brain-damaged donors present ethical problems which are discussed in Sect. 24.3. The anaesthetist responsible for the care of the recipient must take *no* part in the treatment of a brain-damaged donor. If the anaesthetist is initially involved, a request must be made for replacement by another colleague.

### 32.2.2 Recipient

Apart from anaesthesia, the main hazard for the recipient is rejection of the graft by an excessive immune response. The drugs used to depress immune response, azathioprine (Imuran) and corticosteroids, create further hazards. Azathioprine effectively suppresses lymphocytes and other white cells and greatly increases liability to infections. Corticosteroids have a similar effect, but when given together with other immunosuppressive agents, they much reduce the chances of rejection, although when given alone they are quite ineffective.

Hazardous side-effects include delayed healing, gastro-intestinal ulceration and haemorrhage.

### 32.2.3 Anaesthetists

Serum hepatitis (Australia antigen) has caused anxiety amongst staff in renal units. Some renal patients carry the antigen in their bloodstream and staff of renal units are therefore exposed to the virus, especially during dialysis sessions.

If patients are known to carry the Australia antigen, everybody concerned in their treatment should carry out the procedures outlined in Sect. 21.5.2.

### 32.2.4 Timing of Anaesthesia

When the kidney is from a healthy donor the procedures can be done at leisure and at the optimum moment. Brain-damaged donors' kidneys, on the other hand, become available at short notice, but the inevitable delay in tissue typing (3-4 h) gives time for digestion of the last meal and preparatory measures, including the most important cross-matching of 2 units of blood.

### 32.2.5 Pre-operative Preparation

Patients selected for transplantation are on regular dialysis and living at home, so presumably they are in reasonable physical condition. In recent years, the care and health of patients in chronic renal failure has improved immensely. Hypertension is usually under control and chronic anaemia well compensated.

Patients must have recently received dialysis, for this reduces chances of rejection. Blood potassium should not be more than 5 mmol/l, so Hartmann's solution is unsuitable in chronic renal failure.

### 32.2.6 Anaesthetic Room Procedures

Mention has been made of susceptibility to infection of patients receiving immunosuppressive therapy.

All anaesthetic procedures should be undertaken with presterilised equipment, which is kept ready in a prepared pack in the operating theatre or anaesthetic room. This pack should contain sterile gown, gloves and towel and a sterile anaesthetic circuit, in addition to all the other items an anaesthetist could be expected to require.

Corticosteroids such as methylprednisolone sodium succinate (Solu-Medrone) and azathioprine and frusemide (Lasix) should also be included for administration before, during and after anaesthesia in accordance with the surgeon's instructions.

It is usual to set up two separate infusion sets connected with a Y-piece, one containing normal saline, which is used for administration of the immunosuppressive agents, and the other for fluid replacement by dextrose saline. Optional ancillary equipment includes an electrocardiograph monitor and central venous pressure line. The latter is non-essential and those without experience should avoid its use.

### 32.2.7 Anaesthetic Techniques

Premedication is a matter of personal preference and there is no reason to change from the usual routine.

Regional (subdural and epidural) methods have been used with satisfactory results in North America. Bleeding is reduced, hypertension controlled and relaxed vessels facilitate sutures. Additional light sedation is routine. Since these procedures block the neuro-endocrine response to injury, including secretion of antidiuretic hormone, a reduction of immunological response is possible.

In the United Kingdom, however, there is preference for general anaesthesia and a variety of methods have been used, all apparently successful.

Whatever technique is chosen, the reduced oxygen-carrying capacity of patients is a reason for extra care in avoiding hypoxic episodes due to laryngeal spasm. Five minutes' pre-induction oxygenation is a rule in many units.

As renal transplantation is an extraperitoneal procedure, profound relaxation and tracheal intubation are not essential. The operation could be successfully carried out with an oral airway and an inhalational agent such as halothane. Sudden hypotension has been recorded as a drawback of this method, but this probably arose from too great a depth of anaesthesia prior to surgical incision. Most British anaesthetists prefer an intravenous induction followed by a relaxant, intubation, and maintenance with nitrous oxide and oxygen and an inhalational supplement, usually controlling ventilation.

Care needs to be exercised in the use of relaxants. Suxamethonium can increase serum potassium and repeated doses are best avoided, although an initial dose for intubation is acceptable, with maintenance for relaxation by a non-depolarising agent other than curare, which is partially excreted by the kidney, and gallamine, which is totally dependent upon a functioning kidney. If suxamethonium is used initially, application of cricoid pressure is recommended in case of regurgitation of residual stomach contents. Pancuronium and fazadinium are free from these drawbacks. Of supplementary inhalational agents, methoxyflurane is best avoided, owing to its potential nephrotoxicity. Halothane has the advantage of controlling hypertension and bleeding, which can be troublesome in lightly anaesthetised patients, and provides smooth anaesthesia whilst reducing the overall dose of relaxants.

Careful measurement of blood loss and accurate replacement is important to avoid overload of the circulation, always allowing for blood lost on drapes and gowns.

## 32.3  Bladder and Prostate

The position of the bladder and prostate in the lower abdomen make spinal and epidural analgesia very acceptable methods to surgeons, because relaxation is excellent and bleeding minimal. This is of particular value for transurethral resection. Intravenous infusions should always be set up before carrying out either procedure.

Controlled hypotension is a popular technique for retropubic prostatectomy (see Chap. 19). In elderly subjects, reduced bleeding can often be achieved by controlled respiration and halothane. Whichever method is used, the blood pressure should be allowed to rise before the bladder is closed, to give an opportunity to deal with any bleeding points which may appear, and prevent reactionary haemorrhage. Large doses of muscle relaxants are not necessary for bladder and prostate surgery, since the peritoneum is never opened.

### 32.3.1  Cystoscopy

Cystoscopy is the commonest urological procedure and precedes all operations on the bladder. Local analgesia with 1%-2% lignocaine is satisfactory, especially in females. In the United Kingdom general anaesthesia is more usual, but it is not always easy to carry out smoothly.The chief problem is coughing, laryngospasm and hiccup, since many patients who suffer from carcinoma of the bladder are heavy smokers with chronic cough. They are unsuitable for unpremedicated anaesthesia in a day unit (see Chap. 46).

An antispasmodic medication such as promethazine with pethidine should always be given and sufficient thiopentone to allow absorption of enough nitrous oxide, oxygen and halothane to subdue the cough reflex before its effect wears off. Addition of a little carbon dioxide helps to achieve a more rapid rise in blood concentration of halothane.

### 32.3.2  Bladder Resection

Carcinoma of the bladder requires surgery either for partial excision and implantation of radium, or for total cystectomy and implantation of the ureters into a preformed ileal pouch or the sigmoid colon.

Partial cystectomy is a straightforward procedure, but total cyst-ectomy presents problems. Patients have usually received radiotherapy, so the bladder has become fixed, fibrosed and surrounded by vascular adhesions. Profuse haemorrhage occurs during removal, even though the internal iliac arteries on either side have been ligated. Rapid infusion of blood or other fluid under pressure is always necessary until the surgeon can identify and secure the major bleeding sites. A double intravenous infusion is sometimes put up for rapid blood replacement. The operation takes more than 4 h, but more than half of this time is spent creating the ileal pouch. During this time, as in gastric surgery, the surgical stimulus is minimal and respiration can be controlled under light anaesthesia without additional relaxant. Alternatively, spontaneous respiration is practicable at this stage, until closure of the peritoneum, for which addition of a little relaxant or further anaesthetic becomes necessary.

# 33 Orthopaedic Surgery

Orthopaedic surgery divides itself into emergencies arising from trauma from industrial, domestic or road traffic accidents, and elective surgery, mainly aimed at correction of deformities caused by disease of bone and joints. The anaesthetic hazards of the two divisions vary accordingly.

## 33.1 Emergencies

Orthopaedic emergencies carry the same hazards of anaesthesia as for other emergency conditions, particularly that of a full stomach, which are set out in detail in Part III.

### 33.1.1 Shock

Traumatic and haemorrhagic shock is always present to some extent and is often intensified by the victims' anxieties, particularly if they are wage-earners and have a family to support or if they are self-employed and have their own business to consider. This class of patient benefits on admission from a tranquilliser as well as an opiate drug to control pain, e.g. pethidine and chlorpromazine or phenoperidine and droperidol combined with an intravenous infusion, pending group and cross-matching of blood if surgery is contemplated.

Abdominal and thoracic injuries frequently accompany major accidents, and at the pre-anaesthetic examination anaesthetists should consult with surgeons about the possibility of laparotomy or thoracotomy in addition to treatment of any fractures. Anaesthesia can then be planned accordingly, allowing for intubation with full relaxation and assurance that blood will be available for resuscitation, or if that is impossible, fresh frozen plasma, dextran 70 or Hartmann's solution, in that order of preference.

Reference has already been made to the treatment of traumatic and haemorrhagic shock in Chap. 26. Injured patients who require diagnostic X-ray often return to the accident and emergency department needing resuscitation before going to the theatre. In any case, anaesthesia for major accidents should never begin on a shocked patient, and resuscitation should be continued until a good peripheral circulation returns and a systolic blood pressure of 12 kPa is reached. Experience some years ago showed that patients receiving pethidine, chlorpromazine and intravenous infusion on admission to accident and emergency departments never needed resuscitation after returning from the X-ray department, and urine was always obtained on catheterisation. This compared with a control series receiving opiates only, and an intravenous infusion, in whom resuscitation on return from the X-ray department was always needed and from whom no urine was ever obtained on catheterisation.

Anaesthetic techniques are a matter of personal choice, but whatever method is used a careful watch must be kept during operation for blood loss and allowance of up to 50% of the measured loss made for blood on towels, operating gowns and theatre floor, especially during operations on the femur or during laparotomy for abdominal haemorrhage.

### 33.1.2 Stove-in Chest

Multiple rib fractures are not uncommon after road traffic accidents. As explained in Chap. 40, paradoxical respiration and cardiovascular and respiratory distress are usually present. The incidence of paradox is greater and more severe with posterior fractures of the ribs than with anterior. In addition to routine resuscitation, severe paradox will require immediate intubation and mechanical inflation with 100% oxygen. Suggestions for assessing indications for mechanical ventilation are set out in Chap. 24.

Subsequent treatment varies. If the trachea or bronchus is ruptured (as shown by an air leak on inflation) or other intrathoracic injury suspected, a general anaesthetic for thoracotomy and internal fixation of fractured ribs by wiring may be attempted (a long and tedious procedure). Anaesthesia should be as for any thoracotomy, bearing in mind the need for suction of the trachea to remove any blood.

If there is no indication for thoracotomy, most units prefer to treat multiple rib fractures by mechanical ventilation through a tracheostomy.

In the early stage, areas of collapsed lung and bronchospasm require high inflation pressures, possibly higher than the ventilator can produce, necessitating manual inflation for the first few hours. Subsequent treatment is the same for any patient receiving mechanical ventilation (see Chap. 24).

### 33.1.3  Hip Fractures

Fractures of the femoral neck receive treatment as emergencies in many units, in the interest of early mobility and avoidance of pulmonary complications and deep vein thrombosis. Possibly an additional reason is to avoid overloading orthopaedic theatre lists planned for the following day.

Femoral neck fractures are almost exclusively the prerogative of old age. The fall causing the fracture may be the result of a syncopal attack or of weakness from an acute infection, either respiratory or urinary.

Such patients require careful clinical examination before anaesthesia to exclude such disorders. Estimation of red cell and haemoglobin levels, as well as electrocardiographic and chest X-ray examinations should precede surgery, together with intravenous therapy to reverse dehydration, electrolyte imbalance or anaemia (see Chap. 20).

Any simple anaesthetic technique with light premedication is sufficient. Intubation is optional. If an image intensifier is available, the operative time for hip nailing can be as short as 5 min and that for pin and plating 45 min instead of 1.5 h.

## 33.2  Elective Surgery

In progressive order of severity, routine orthopaedic procedures can be classified as follows:

1) *Minor.* Manipulations and plastic procedures on feet and hands

2) *Moderate.* Open reduction and fixation of fractures, and procedures to correct deformity and increase stability, such as arthrodesis and tendon transplantation

3) *Major.* Hip replacement, operations on the spine (laminectomy and fusion), and operations to correct scoliosis

### 33.2.1  Minor and Moderate Procedures

For manipulations a single dose of thiopentone is adequate; for other procedures it should be supplemented with nitrous oxide and intravenous analgesic or an inhalational agent (trichloroethylene is very useful). Since the skin is more sensitive than underlying muscle, absence of reaction to skin incision indicates adequate depth of anaesthesia, which indeed can subsequently be lightened. The impression of some surgeons that a muscle relaxant helps to lengthen muscles contracted after displaced fractures is not correct and muscle relaxants should not be used for such purposes.

### 33.2.2  Hip Replacement

In recent years hip replacement has become a common major orthopaedic procedure. Patients are usually aged 60 years or more and electrocardiographic examination may reveal old coronary artery disease. Pre-operative preparation should include treatment of anaemia, if present, and of chronic respiratory infection. Recent coronary infarct (Sect. 2.3.1) is an indication for 6 months' postponement of the operation. In spite of the extensive trauma and blood loss and the age of the patient, results are good and restoration of mobility justifies an occasional risk. Sometimes the question of bilateral replacement arises and whilst some hesitate it is being undertaken successfully with increased frequency. In favour, it is argued that two separate operations expose the patient to double hazards of postoperative complications, especially pulmonary embolism. Reasonably rapid surgery and careful fluid replacement help to ensure good results. Two main hazards are blood loss and the hypotensive effects of methylmethacrylate, the basis of the cement used to bond metal prostheses to bone.

Blood loss should always be measured; it will be between 500 and 1500 ml, depending partly on the anaesthetic technique and partly on the extent of arthritic changes. During the first 24 h after operation, loss varies between 500 and 1000 ml, for which replacement should be made. Intravenous infusion should begin with some electrolyte combination (Hartmann's or dextrose saline) running freely, followed by blood as soon as the surgeon begins to prepare the acetabulum, which involves removal of osteophytes and fibrous tissue by a process known as reaming and is associated with particularly free loss of blood.

The solvent for the acrylic cement, methylmethacrylate, if absorbed into the bloodstream can cause hypotension. In the early days, severe hypotension during the insertion of cement into the femoral shaft was sometimes reported. Adverse incidents are rarer since adoption of the practice of venting the femoral shaft with a small plastic tube to allow vapour to escape. Accurate blood replacement, which compensates for any vasodilating action of the monomer in the acrylate, may be another preventive factor.

*Regional Analgesia.* Subdural (spinal) analgesia with light sedation gives excellent results, reducing blood loss and operative shock.

*General Anaesthesia.* Any routine method of general anaesthetic is acceptable. Most anaesthetists intubate (but this is by no means essential) and maintain a light general anaesthesia with a relaxant and controlled ventilation by a mechanical ventilator. Anaesthesia is maintained by nitrous oxide and oxygen, supplemented by an analgesic such as pethidine or the neuroleptic combination of droperidol and fentanyl, or by 0.5%-1% halothane.

Premedication with 50 mg each of chlorpromazine and pethidine, followed by the same dose given intravenously and 150-200 mg thiopentone, anaesthesia being maintained with an oral airway, spontaneous respiration and 1% halothane, gives good results. A small initial fall in blood pressure after the chlorpromazine is reversed by speeding up the intravenous infusion, and the stimulus of surgery is an immediate restorative.

Blood loss is reduced, seldom exceeding 500 ml. Postoperative recovery, although slower than with other techniques, is notably free from restlessness and fluctuations of systolic blood pressure. The 24-h urine output exceeds 1000 ml in all patients, and they appear fresh and relaxed the following day.

### 33.2.3 Laminectomy

Laminectomy (removal of the lamina of the vertebrae) is undertaken by orthopaedic surgeons for removal of the prolapsed nucleus of inter-vertebral discs causing pressure on nerves and by neurosurgeons for removal of spinal tumours. Subjects are often young and active.

The anaesthetic hazards of the operation arise from the position of the patient and the blood loss.

*Positioning the Patient.* The operation may be undertaken with the patient in either the prone or the lateral position. The hazards of the prone position have been mentioned in Chap. 15. Careful positioning is vital and anaesthetists must make sure there is no pressure on the abdomen with congestion of the venous system, especially the spinal veins. Most anaesthetists prefer the lateral position.

*Blood Loss.* Blood loss can be deceptive. Although obvious during the early part of the operation, during exposure of lamina it becomes less obvious from the deeper parts of the wound from which blood is removed by suction. A careful watch on the contents of the suction bottle gives a good idea of any hidden blood loss.

Haemorrhage can be kept to a minimum and the operation shortened by smooth anaesthesia and use of controlled hypotension (see Chap. 19). Hyperventilation with halothane alone provides an acceptable operative field. The rise of venous pressure after coughing is particularly obvious in this operation. Even at a systolic pressure of 10.7 kPa the wound fills with venous blood, after coughing or straining.

*Anaesthetic Technique.* Endotracheal anaesthesia is essential. A controlled hypotensive technique with moderate head-down tilt to protect the cerebral circulation improves venous drainage and ensures a dry operative field.

### 33.2.4 Spinal Fusion

Immobilisation of the vertebral column with bone grafts is undertaken either separately or in conjunction with laminectomy. The anaesthetic problems do not differ from those already mentioned.

### 33.2.5 Correction of Scoliosis

Procedures to correct scoliosis require highly specialised surgical and anaesthetic techniques and are best avoided by junior anaesthetists. In addition to excessive blood loss, pneumothorax is a likely complication. Postoperative care in an intensive care unit with mechanical ventilation is usual.

## 33.3  Tourniquets

Failure to remove a tourniquet is a hazard common to all orthopaedic operations on limbs. Although anaesthetists supervise their application, surgeons are responsible for removal.

A stout piece of rubber tubing applied over a towel to the lower limb is no longer tolerated as a tourniquet. Besides causing damage to skin and blood vessels, removal can easily be overlooked at the end of the operation.

An inflatable cuff like that used for blood pressure estimation is used for tourniquets on the upper limbs. This avoids damage to the musculo-spinal or radial nerves. After applying the cuff and before inflation, the arm is exsanguinated by holding it vertically for a few minutes, followed by application of an Esmarch bandage from the fingers to the lower end of the cuff, after which the cuff should be inflated to 3 or 4 kPa above pre-operative blood pressure and the Esmarch bandage removed. Leaky cuffs are common; periodical additional inflation may be required.

The most satisfactory tourniquet for upper or lower limbs is an inflatable cuff attached to an apparatus which maintains a constant pressure by evaporation of a cylinder of liquid (the Kidde appliance).

If this is not available for lower limbs, then an Esmarch bandage carefully applied over a cotton towel at the upper extent of the thigh is satisfactory, preceded by exsanguination as described for the arm.

Care should be taken that the cuff or bandage is as high up into the groin as possible, otherwise fibres of the quadriceps muscle may be torn when the knee is flexed for operations for internal derangements of the knee or removal of the patella.

The time of application of the tourniquet should be recorded.

The time of release of tourniquet depends on local practice. Some units will not leave a tourniquet on for more than 1 h and others will tolerate up to 2 h. The decision is a matter for the surgeon.

Tourniquet application is a painful procedure and first-plane anaes-thesia should be induced beforehand. After being applied for 20 min, lack of oxygen begins to impair nerve conduction and pain sensation is reduced, returning rapidly on release of the tourniquet when, if anaesthesia is too light, movements of the limbs may occur.

Failure to remove a tourniquet at the end of an operation has already been mentioned. Disasters have occurred even in spite of bitter com-plaints of pain and discomfort by patients.

It is impossible to leave a Kidde tourniquet inflated if the inflating device is fixed to a drip stand. If an Esmarch bandage is used in its place, it must be secured to the operating table in such a way that the patient cannot be removed from the table with the tourniquet still applied.

# 34 Neurosurgery

Neurosurgical operations can be divided rather arbitrarily into those performed supratentorially and those performed subtentorially.

## 34.1 Local Analgesia for Supratentorial Operations

Satisfactory operating conditions for certain operations can be provided under local analgesia and indeed local analgesia is preferred:

1) For the creation of burr holes through the skull to reduce intra-cranial pressure, particularly in head injuries

2) If it is necessary for the patient to be conscious at some subsequent stage of the operation

3) In certain emergencies which already have a dangerous rate of rise of intracranial pressure, e.g. middle meningeal haemorrhage

4) If for any other reason general anaesthesia is contra-indicated

As premedication, phenobarbitone 200 mg intramuscularly or diazepam 10 mg intravenously gives satisfactory sedation for local analgesia. Opiates should be avoided because of their potential

respiratory depressant effect. Procedures under local analgesia do not
make the presence of an anaesthetist unnecessary: one should always be
present to watch for changes in vital signs, including changes in
consciousness, and to reassure the patient during the procedure. The
method is obviously unsuitable for children and for unco-operative,
irritable, or semiconscious patients.

## 34.2  General Anaesthesia for Supratentorial Operations

### 34.2.1  Premedication
When intracranial pressure is known to be high or there is a head injury,
sedative premedication should be avoided, in spite of anxiety on the part
of the patient. Atropine or hyoscine are necessary as drying agents,
and inclusion of beta blockers in the premedication has been recommended in order to reduce the hypertensive response to intubation.

Fully conscious patients benefit from a small dose of morphine
(10 mg) or heroin (2.5 mg). If, for any reason, opiates are considered
undesirable, a tranquillising agent such as a phenothiazine derivative
(chlorpromazine or promethazine 25-50 mg) is an adequate substitute
and has useful antispasm and beta-blocking action, in addition to
sedative properties.

### 34.2.2  Induction
Thiopentone (which reduces intracranial pressure) should be used for
induction, followed by a relaxant dose of suxamethonium and generous
spraying of trachea and larynx with 4% lignocaine before passage of the
largest flexible endotracheal tube the larynx will allow. Vigorous hyperventilation should follow and a dose of a long-acting relaxant such as
curare or pancuronium be administered as soon as there are signs that the
effects of the suxamethonium are wearing off. Since at this stage
coughing or straining results in congestion of the brain, which lasts for a
considerable time, the long-acting relaxant should be given sooner rather
than later.

### 34.2.3  Maintenance
Maintenance of anaesthesia can be carried out in one of two ways, either
hyperventilation with nitrous oxide, oxygen and supplementary
intermittent injections of a neuroleptanalgesic drug, fentanyl, phenoperidine or droperidol; or hyperventilation with inhalational agents in
modest concentrations, such as 0.5%-1.0% halothane.

Halothane has the theoretical disadvantage that it increases cerebral
blood flow, which is contra-indicated in the presence of oedema. Nevertheless, results are satisfactory because hyperventilation reduces brain
volume, neutralising any increase due to halothane.

The neuroleptanalgesic drugs reduce intracranial pressure only in large doses which may cause unwelcome respiratory depression during recovery. Too small doses of analgesic supplements may result in hypertensive responses to surgical stimulus, neutralising any reduction of intracranial pressure which may have been achieved. The neurolept technique should only be used by those familiar with it in other fields.

## 34.3  Subtentorial Operations

In addition to the problems already set out for supratentorial lesions, subtentorial lesions have further hazards.

Obstruction of the flow of cerebrospinal fluid can cause hydrocephalus, with 'coning' of the cerebellum into the foramen magnum, and cardiovascular and respiratory disturbances.

Also, the operation is performed in unusual positions which present additional anaesthetic problems.

The patients may be either adults or children. Adults are often ill, undernourished and dehydrated from vomiting. Children, on the other hand, are usually in good shape.

### 34.3.1  Premedication
Opiates, being respiratory depressants, are contra-indicated. The drying action of atropine is necessary and phenobarbitone or chlorpromazine in an appropriate dose is acceptable as premedication for children and adults, and provides sedation for these anxious patients.

### 34.3.2  Positioning of Patient
The position for surgery may be either prone (face down), sitting, or the lateral semiprone position sometimes known as the 'Manchester' or 'park bench' position.

The prone position is the least suitable because it interferes with venous return from the lower limbs and causes congestion of the posterior spinal veins. Flexion of the head (a surgical requirement) increases the bleeding from the skull.

The prone position has been replaced by the sitting position, which carries a considerable risk of hypotension especially during the early part of the operation, or the modified lateral semiprone position with a slight head-up tilt and lateral rotation of the table to improve access which overcomes the disadvantages of the prone and sitting positions.

### 34.3.3  Anaesthetic Technique
Because operations on the posterior fossa carry a serious risk of cardiovascular complications and respiratory failure, many anaesthetists prefer to maintain spontaneous respiration instead of controlled breathing.

There has recently, however, been a shift in favour of controlled respiration, relying on circulatory rather than respiratory signs to indicate disturbances of sensitive areas in the brain stem.

With spontaneous breathing it is difficult to avoid coughing on the tube without supplementary halothane, which can cause hypotensive problems in the sitting position.

### 34.3.4 Accidental Endobronchial Intubation

Endotracheal intubation takes place with the head extended; when the head is flexed before surgery, the end of the endotracheal tube can be pushed down the trachea and has on occasions entered the right main bronchus. When this happens the occluded lung is not aerated, a right-to-left circulatory shunt develops, with accumulation of carbon dioxide and falling oxygen tension. The brain size increases and unless the error is diagnosed and rectified death may easily follow. It can be prevented by careful estimation of the length of the tube required by placing it outside the neck of the patient with the tip in the suprasternal notch and cutting the end of the tube level with the mouth. Children are particularly at risk and a tube should be selected which does not pass more than 2.5 cm beyond the larynx.

### 34.3.5 Disturbance of Vital Functions

Cardiac irregularities, fluctuations in blood pressure, tachycardia or bradycardia are all encountered during subtentorial procedures. Tachycardia is often encountered with hydrocephalus and subsides after tapping the ventricle to reduce pressure.

Traction on the sensory root of the fifth nerve during mobilisation of acoustic neuromata causes hypertension which may be masked by halothane. Traction on vagal roots causes bradycardia and hypotension (which can to a considerable extent be prevented by atropine). Extreme variations of pulse and blood pressure are of serious prognostic significance; the surgeon should be warned since persistence with surgery in the area responsible can lead to death.

Postural hypotension usually occurs early in anaesthesia in the sitting position, and is not accompanied by any rise in pulse rate. If pressure falls the rate of infusion should be increased to administer up to 500 ml of fluid in 10 min, which should restore pressure to an acceptable level. If that is not successful, a small dose of an intravenous vasopressor (5 mg methoxamine) should restore blood pressure to a normal level. If this fails, the patient must be put into the horizontal position as soon as possible (not a popular movement with the surgeon).

### 34.3.6 Air Embolus

The sitting position gives rise to subatmospheric pressure in the infra-cranial veins, increasing the risk of air embolism during the surgical approach through cut vessels in the suboccipital venous plexus, or even a tear in the lateral sinus.

Air embolus should be suspected if a sudden fall in blood pressure of 1.3 kPa or an increase in pulse rate of 10 beats per minute occurs for which there is no explanation. The appearance of a little froth from one of the veins in the operative area, after pressure on the internal jugular veins, will confirm the diagnosis.

Better known signs such as the 'millwheel murmur' over the heart occur late and are of poor prognostic significance.

Early identification and closure of the exposed vein will restore stability after small emboli. If blood pressure continues to fall after this, rapid intravenous infusion and vasopressors should be effective, but if pressure falls to 9.3 kPa and does not respond to any of the above measures within 2-3 min, the sitting position should be abandoned, the patient put in the lateral position and treatment carried out as for air embolus as outlined in Sect. 21.4.3.

## 34.4  Head Injuries

Patients with head injuries are often admitted to hospitals without neuro-surgical facilities. The duty anaesthetist is responsible for pre-anaesthetic assessment, for treatment of airway problems associated with unconsciousness or for treatment of haemorrhage. The situation abounds with hazards, both initially and subsequently should anaesthesia be required.

### 34.4.1  Initial Hazards
On admission patients may present:

1) Unconscious, with oxygen lack and carbon dioxide accumulation, from airway problems caused by respiratory obstruction.

2) With haemorrhagic shock from wounds elsewhere compromising cerebral circulation.

3) With associated injuries. These are present in 30% of cases of which 8% are serious. Fractured ribs, ruptured liver, spleen, bowel or kidney may exacerbate the shock already produced by haemorrhage.

### 34.4.2  Preliminary Treatment
*Care of Airway.* Unconscious patients should be turned into the lateral position, the pharynx cleared of secretions by suction, an oral airway inserted and oxygen administered. Failure of these simple measures to clear the airway indicates need for endotracheal intubation under local analgesia. A stomach tube should be passed to empty the stomach.

*Acute Haemorrhagic Shock.* An intravenous infusion should be set up as soon as possible and blood taken for grouping and cross-matching. If resuscitative treatment to reverse the signs of shock fails, a careful reexamination of the patient should be made for alternative causes of shock, e.g. internal injuries.

*Assessment of Level of Consciousness.* The level of consciousness varies considerably in patients with head injuries. Some patients who are unconscious on admission recover but subsequently subside again into unconsciousness. This syndrome is diagnostic either of a subdural haematoma or increasing cerebral oedema both of which require urgent treatment.

In order to monitor the level of consciousness, some charting method is helpful, recording the state of the eyes and orientation and co-ordination in terms of motor and verbal response to stimuli. A sample chart is shown in Fig. 3.

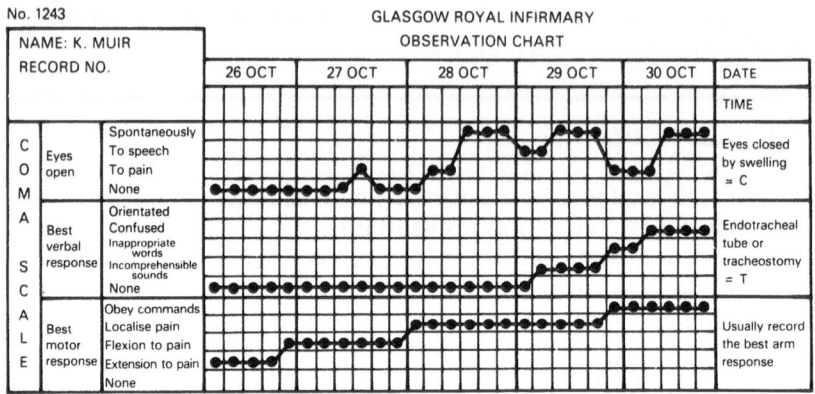

**Fig. 3.** Coma chart for bedside recording. Five motor responses are included in this simplified scale; abnormal flexion is recorded as 'flexion'. (Permission of Editor, Journal of the Royal College of Physicians, London.)

### 34.4.3  Anaesthesia

An authority on anaesthesia for head injuries has remarked that 'the patient with a recent severe closed head injury is perhaps more at risk from the activities of the anaesthetist than any other neurosurgical patient'. The reasons for this statement are:

1) Unless there is an open fracture, internal head injuries are associated with severe cerebral compression and associated disorder of blood flow.

2) Further damage to the brain can follow the use of volatile agents which increase blood flow or the accumulation of carbon dioxide, or coughing and straining which increases congestion and swelling.

3) Cerebral oedema may persist following head injuries for up to a week, reaching its maximum about 36 h after injury.

Dehydrating fluids are not indicated since they increase blood volume and thus increase rather than decrease oedema. Hydrocortisone 4 mg intramuscularly 4-6 hourly is a popular remedy but its effectiveness has not been fully established; 50 mg chlorpromazine intramuscularly or intravenously 8-hourly has had advocates in the past, particularly for brain stem injuries.

Concussion should not be treated lightly. Concussed patients requiring anaesthesia should be treated as cases of major head injury, because they are susceptible to cerebral oedema which may not become evident until 36 h after the injury.

*Skull Fractures.* Surgery may be required for elevation of the fractured segment. Usually local analgesia is sufficient.

*Subdural Haematoma.* Treatment may be confined to the creation of burr holes under local analgesia to reduce pressure, or decompression under general anaesthesia by turning down a bone flap and removal of the haematoma.

Although unconscious at the outset, the patient may recover consciousness during the operation when the pressure of clot is released. Even with local analgesia, recovery of consciousness may be associated with cerebral irritation and restlessness.

It is advisable in such circumstances to anticipate return of consciousness by passing an endotracheal tube after spraying larynx and trachea with 4% lignocaine before surgery. Should consciousness return, restlessness can then be controlled by light inhalational anaesthesia.

General anaesthesia for head injuries does not differ significantly from that described for supratentorial lesions, except that some surgeons do not encourage the use of halothane because it may increase cerebral oedema.

As an alternative, patients are paralysed with curare, receiving a further 10 mg every hour, anaesthesia being maintained with nitrous oxide and oxygen and a supplement of 0.1 mg thiopentone half-hourly to reduce cerebral blood flow. Often the first person to notice lack of relaxation and return of muscle power is the neurosurgeon who may complain that the brain has become 'tight'.

### 34.4.4 Postoperative Care

Neurosurgical patients should spend the first 24 h after operation in an intensive care unit. Those requiring respiratory support are referred to the anaesthetic department. The problems of prolonged treatment with ventilators are discussed in Chap. 24.

# 35 Ear, Nose and Throat and Maxillofacial Surgery

Although problems of microsurgery of the ear differ somewhat from those encountered in operations on nose and throat, the latter have much in common with maxillofacial injuries and plastic correction of nasal defects, which are therefore included in this chapter.

## 35.1 Middle Ear

### 35.1.1 Myringotomy

Incision of the eardrum for acutely inflamed middle ear followed by the insertion of a grommet drain is most commonly undertaken in children. The eardrum is exquisitely sensitive, especially when acutely inflamed.

Reflex cardiac arrest can occur during myringotomy in apprehensive children, with a high level of circulating adrenaline, if they are not fully anaesthetised.

The classical signs of third-stage, first-plane anaesthesia must be evident before allowing the surgeon to proceed. The surgeon will tolerate delay when it is in the interests of safety. As the operation is short, endotracheal intubation is not necessary.

## 35.1.2  Microsurgery

Operations on the middle ear using the operating microscope include myringoplasty, stapedectomy and mastoidectomy. In all these conditions the anaesthetic technique chosen should be one which reduces oozing of blood into the operative field which slows up the operation and at times makes it almost impossible. At the same time, anaesthetic techniques should ensure a calm postoperative recovery in which tinnitus, vertigo and nausea are minimal.

Premedication with an anti-emetic, preferably a phenothiazine derivative, and pethidine contributes to smooth anaesthesia, minimising nausea and vertigo during recovery.

There are various ways of securing a dry operative field. Anaesthesia should be of sufficient depth to avoid coughing on the tube when the surgeon positions the head under the microscope just before the start of the operation. Coughing on the tube at this moment produces congestion in the middle ear which can take up to half an hour to subside. The use of a long-acting relaxant with hyperventilation and halothane anaesthesia are the most certain ways of avoiding these hazards.

Elevation of head and trunk (reverse Trendelenburg) reduces congestion, especially if vasodilator agents are used to ensure good venous drainage. If a table which splits in the middle is available there is no need to lower the legs; this allows greater elevation of the trunk without unacceptable fall in blood pressure.

For many years the author has used the following method to produce a dry field: After light premedication with pethidine and promethazine, an intravenous injection of 50 mg pethidine, promethazine and chlorpromazine in 20 ml saline is given slowly until the patient drops into a light sleep. A sleep dose of thiopentone with an adequate dose of relaxant follows, and after intubation anaesthesia is maintained with nitrous oxide, oxygen and halothane in approximately 1% concentration. With elevation of the trunk as already described, a dry operative field results, often with the blood pressure in excess of 13 kPa. This technique avoids the need for controlled hypotension and ensures almost entire freedom from nausea, tinnitus and vertigo on the day after operation.

Controlled hypotension with posture is a popular way of ensuring dry operative fields (see Chap. 19). The need to raise the head increases the risk of reducing cerebral circulation, especially in elderly patients with inelastic blood vessels. Results are good in experienced hands, but the method should be avoided by the inexperienced.

A real hazard of anaesthesia for middle ear surgery is the effect on concentration of tedium and monotony. The surgeon has a monopoly of the operative field and for most of the operation the anaesthetist remains in complete ignorance of what is happening (unless of course the field is congested, when he soon knows all about it). This predisposes to sleepiness. An occasional cup of coffee is recommended to relieve tedium and refresh concentration, whilst not interfering with supervision of the patient.

## 35.2  Nose and Mouth

The main hazard of surgery of nose, maxilla, frontal sinus, etc., is aspiration of blood and foreign material into the respiratory tract during or after operation. Anaesthetic techniques should be chosen which avoid such hazards.

### 35.2.1  Premedication
To reduce laryngospasm and vomiting during recovery, premedication should include antitussive and anti-emetic agents which do not depress respiration. A combination of antihistamines, preferably phenothiazine derivatives, with small doses of pethidine is satisfactory.

### 35.2.2  Vasoconstriction
Pretreatment with cocaine paste or a vasodilator spray will reduce bleeding during operation only if sufficient time is allowed for them to become maximally effective, i.e. about 15-20 min after application of paste or spray in the anaesthetic room before induction of anaesthesia.

### 35.2.3  Avoiding Congestion
The need to avoid congestion from coughing during positioning for the operation is just as great as during anaesthesia for middle ear surgery. The same precautions, therefore, apply.

### 35.2.4  Intubation
Intubation is by the oral route for surgery of the nose and sinuses but the nasal route is essential for procedures in the mouth and on the tongue. A cuffed tube can be used for either route, in either case a paraffin impregnated gauze throat pack should be placed in position before operation, to absorb blood in the pharynx, preventing accumulation and inhalation should the endotracheal cuff collapse.

### 35.2.5  Maintenance
Halothane is suitable for maintenance of anaesthesia and should not be withdrawn too soon at the end of the operation. A head-up position during surgery as described for middle ear surgery reduces venous congestion.

### 35.2.6  Extubation
If anaesthesia is too light at the end of operation, coughing and spasm on extubation will increase oozing and haematoma formation: unwelcome to the surgeon. Alternatively, if anaesthesia is too deep, removal of the tube will leave the larynx unprotected against inhalation of blood. Anaesthetists have to steer a middle course erring on the side of depth but should insist on a head-down position with suction under direct vision.

Blood often accumulates in the posterior nasal space and unless sought for may be missed. Once the pharynx and posterior nasal space appear clear of blood, the patient can be turned on the side (still keeping the head down), the endotracheal tube removed and an oral airway inserted whilst maintaining gentle suction of the pharynx.

## 35.3  Maxillofacial Surgery

Maxillofacial injuries are common after road traffic accidents. Airway problems are commonplace with fractured jaws or maxillae or injuries to the tongue. Haemorrhage and injuries elsewhere increase the likelihood of haemorrhagic shock, whilst associated head injuries result in disordered consciousness, not always evident on admission.

### 35.3.1  Pre-anaesthetic Care

The principal hazard being airway obstruction, anaesthetic care even before operation must concentrate on ways and means of ensuring unobstructed respiration.

On arrival in the anaesthetic room the patient should lie supine in a head-down position to avoid inhalation of blood. Anaesthetist and surgeon should jointly examine the patient, inspecting the extent of injury in the mouth. A piece of gauze round the tongue is a help. in bringing it forward to allow examination of fauces and pharynx. Palpation of the mandible will reveal the presence of a fracture. When present, of course, this will prevent maintenance of airway by drawing the jaw forward, and is overcome by traction on a suture through the posterior third of the tongue. When blood clot and debris have been cleared away an oral airway should be inserted to prevent recurrence of obstruction, preferably after a 4% lignocaine spray to the pharynx to help tolerance. If for any reason (e.g. severe laceration of the tongue) it appears that maintenance of any airway during induction will be difficult or impossible, endotracheal intubation may have to be carried out with the patient conscious. Injection of intravenous diazepam 10 mg or pethidine, or promethazine 25-30 mg in 5 ml saline may help tolerance of the procedure. The pharynx, vocal cords and trachea should be sprayed with 4% lignocaine or 5% cocaine before intubation. Bronchotracheal analgesia can be secured by injecting 1-2 ml of 5% cocaine through the cricothyroid membrane. After allowing time for the spray to become effective, a tube may then be passed with the aid of a laryngoscope or, if not possible, directed into the larynx by hand in the following way. The index and little finger of one hand are placed over the epiglottis and the tube passed in between them into the larynx. A gum elastic catheter in the tube is helpful as a direction finder. If all procedures fail, tracheostomy becomes unavoidable.

### 35.3.2  Induction and Maintenance

Although experienced anaesthetists recommend induction with intravenous agents and short-acting relaxants for these conditons, inhalation
induction in the head-down position is safer for the inexperienced as
control of the airway is easier and patients do not resist. This method gives
more time for intubation. If the first attempt fails, it is easy to deepen
anaesthesia to a point where a further attempt can be made. If patients
are paralysed and a tube cannot be inserted at the first attempt, inflation
of the lungs in the presence of fractured jaw, lacerated tongue, etc., can
present practical difficulties.

Once intubation has been successfully completed, maintenance of
anaesthesia presents no additional problems. If not done on admission,
an intravenous infusion should be started.

The hazards at the end of the operation (aspiration of blood, debris,
etc.) are the same as those following surgery of the nose and maxilla,
impacted wisdom teeth, etc., and the procedures already described
should be followed except after fixation of fractured jaws by wired
splints. This procedure presents additional hazards during recovery
because the jaws cannot be opened nor can an airway be inserted.

Before wiring is undertaken, the pharynx should be cleared of all
blood and debris and any packs and swabs removed. Pharyngeal
aspiration must be thorough, making sure that no small clots remain in
the postnasal space or in the sulci between gums and jaws. Anaesthesia
must be maintained deep enough to prevent coughing on the tube. Before
wiring the jaws, a stitch of braided silk should be passed through the
dorsum of the tongue and brought out through a gap between the incisor
teeth to ensure a clear airway during recovery. The naso-endotracheal
tube (routine for these cases) should be left in position during recovery
until the swallowing reflexes return or until the patient can remove it
unaided; an anaesthetist should remain close at hand until recovery of
consciousness. A pair of wire cutters must be available should it become
necessary to cut the wires to relieve obstructed respiration.

Postoperative sedation should include anti-emetics and antitussive
agents, whilst doses of respiratory depressant opiates should be kept as
small as possible. Some recommend DF118 (dihydrocodeine) instead of
pethidine to control pain.

## 35.4  Laryngectomy

Since this operation, involving loss of the power of speech, must generate
considerable psychological tension, liberal prescription of tranquillising
agents is indicated in the preparatory stages.

Apart from the long duration and blood loss, the main problem is
airway maintenance during and after removal of the larynx.

Maintenance of anaesthesia with halothane, nitrous oxide and oxygen is satisfactory, with a moderate head-down tilt to reduce congestion and haemorrhage.

Intravenous injection of chlorpromazine (50 mg) together with 50 mg pethidine immediately prior to induction reduces bleeding and congestion whilst reducing the overall amount of anaesthetic required for the long operation.

Usually the endotracheal tube is changed for a cuffed tracheostomy tube when the larynx is removed. The anaesthetist must have a connector available capable of an airtight junction with the tracheostomy tube. Alternatively the endotracheal tube can be replaced by a larger sterile cuffed nylon-reinforced flexible tube, which can be carried down from the tracheostomy opening over the sternum to the anaesthetic machine, thus preventing endotracheal connections soiling the operative field.

Blood loss is often heavy and should always be measured and generous replacement made, allowing up to 40% for blood on the towels and nurses' and surgeons' gowns.

## 35.5  Laryngoscopy and Microsurgery of the Larynx

Although laryngoscopy and microsurgery can be carried out under local anaesthesia, most patients prefer to be unconscious. The hazards of anaesthesia for these procedures under general anaesthetic include oxygen lack during the procedure and respiratory complications from inhalation of debris and blood afterwards, especially if there is oozing from the operation site. The technique of anaesthesia does not differ from that for bronchoscopy (see Sect. 43.3). Microsurgery of the larynx takes longer than laryngoscopy and therefore the anaesthetist has to arrange for some way of insufflating the lungs through a small-bore endotracheal tube whilst the surgeon carries out the procedure. The presence of a small tube does not interfere with the surgeon. Purpose-made nylon-reinforced flexible tubes (Pollard) have been produced whose distal part is about half (5 mm) the diameter of the proximal part (10 mm). It can be fitted with an adult-size cuff, which can be passed through the larynx and then inflated, allowing mechanical ventilation without interfering with surgery. If such a tube is not available, an alternative method is to induce deep anaesthesia with halothane, pass a small-bore endotracheal tube through which oxygen and halothane can be insufflated, with spontaneous respiration providing sufficient anaesthesia to maintain unconsciousness. Topical lignocaine spray (5%) ensures an insensitive larynx and avoids necessity for deep planes of anaesthesia.

A combination of initial deep anaesthesia and neuroleptanalgesia has also been recommended but appears unnecessarily complex since respiratory depression increases the hazards of oxygen lack.

# 36 Paediatric Surgery

Anaesthesia for children, particularly neonates and infants, is a heavy responsibility and should never be delegated to inexperienced junior staff, even for such minor procedures as circumcision. Neonates and infants require gentle handling and those unfamiliar with such small creatures sometimes find difficulty in airway control and vein puncture.

## 36.1  Preparation

Infants older than 12 h when scheduled for surgery nearly always need correction of electrolyte and fluid balance for which an inexperienced anaesthetist should consult a paediatrician or senior colleague.

Hypoglycaemia is a common occurrence in children aged under four or weighing less than 15.5 kg and can be detected by routine Dextrostix testing. Administration of 10 ml milk/kg body weight up to 300 ml four hours before the operation corrects any tendency to hypoglycaemia and does not delay stomach emptying nor is it associated with vomiting or regurgitation. An alternative is to administer 5% glucose intravenously if an intravenous drip is necessary for other reasons. No child should be deprived of food and drink for more than 8 h before operation and preferably only for 4 h.

## 36.2 Premedication

Infants of less than 10 kg do not require sedation but do need atropine. The dose recommended is 0.15 mg/kg up to a maximum of 0.3 mg. This dose is sufficient to block vagal reflex action without disturbing temperature regulation. In some departments, all children over 6 months of age receive 0.6 mg atropine.

Children older than 2 years usually receive some sedative combination. There is a school of thought however that feels that sedation of children is not necessary if they know what is going to happen to them in the anaesthetic room, but most working anaesthetists agree that some form of sedation is helpful to a child. Good rapport with a child established during pre-operative visits by the anaesthetist will give the child a more confident attitude when the time comes to go the anaesthetic room.

Sedation with tranquillising agents whose qualities have been defined as 'inducing indifference to environment' is useful and logical. Trimeprazine (Vallergan) is popular in a dose of 2-4 mg/kg in a syrup (Vallergan Forte) but should be given at least 2 h before the operation to be really effective. The combination of trimeprazine 2 mg/kg and droperidol 0.2 mg/kg 2 h before ensures amnesia.

Morphine in a dose of 0.2 mg/kg is also recommended but should be omitted before inhalational anaesthesia, since the ensuing respiratory depression makes achievement of adequate depth of anaesthesia very difficult.

## 36.3 Anaesthetic Room

Once a child arrives in the anaesthetic room silence is essential and lights should be dimmed. All traffic through or into the anaesthetic room must be forbidden.

## 36.4 Equipment

Choice of the wrong apparatus can be a major hazard in paediatric anaesthesia, particularly with regard to dead space and resistance to respiration.

The tidal volume of a neonate is as little as 20 ml, and one third of this is physiological dead space. Any addition of dead space will hinder elimination of carbon dioxide and reduce available oxygen with increase of respiratory rate which in infants is already high at about 40 per minute. Neonates tolerate oxygen deprivation badly because their requirement per kilogram is greater than an adult's.

Resistance to breathing is higher in infants because the diameter of the trachea in relation to the size of the lungs is much less than in adults, hence increase in resistance by the presence of even a pop-off valve of an endotracheal tube can interfere with normal oxygenation during spontaneous respiration.

For these reasons, special paediatric apparatus is available and should be used for all children less than 20 kg in weight. All paediatric circuits are based on the Ayre's T-piece principle, in which the fresh gases arrive at the bottom of a metal T-piece, one limb of which connects to a face piece or endotracheal tube and the other to a short piece of corrugated tubing which carries away exhaled gases.

To control respiration, a small bag may be fixed on the end of the corrugated tubing for inflation of the lung; alternatively, a finger placed over the end of the tube can have the same effect.

In order to prevent rebreathing when using this system, the flow rate of fresh gases must be twice the minute volume.

The maximum flow possible is about 8 litres, which makes it suitable for children up to the age of ten, at which age minute volume reaches about 4 litres/min.

Small carbon dioxide absorbers of the Waters type are available, but this technique is not widely used because it increases resistance to respiration. However, points in its favour are minimal heat and moisture loss, both of which are of significance during long procedures. Resistance can be overcome by controlled respiration.

## 36.5 Induction

Experienced paediatric anaesthetists favour intravenous induction with thiopentone 3-4 mg/kg using a very fine 25/26 SWG needle through veins on the dorsum of the hand. The use of the veins on the anterior aspect of the wrist in children is not recommended because it is particularly sensitive. Once the child is anaesthetised, however, these veins can be used for intravenous infusions. Before attempting the injection, the child should be told to expect a 'scratch' and not a prick as a puncture with a very fine needle is almost painless. If no suitable veins are available, it is best not to make a second attempt and resort to inhalational induction.

Before starting an inhalational induction children should never be approached from behind but from the front. If the anaesthetist is in this position, most children will hold the face mask themselves. One method is to give 100% nitrous oxide with the mask a few centimetres from the face until the child becomes drowsy then add oxygen, gradually lowering the mask to the face followed by gradual addition of an inhalational agent. For beginners this technique is preferable to an intravenous induction and relaxants.

## 36.6  Intubation

Intubation of neonates, infants and children is becoming more common than in bygone days when the practice was discouraged because it was hazardous and carried a risk of tracheitis and oedema of the larynx. It is true that tracheitis sometimes followed intubation under deep ether where an inspiratory tug could cause inflammatory changes by friction of the tube on the trachea. Oedema of the larynx has occurred as part of generalised oedema in children who have received excessive amounts of sodium in normal saline. Modern fluid therapy has removed the incidence of such an unwelcome complication. Relaxants, controlled respiration and non-irritant tubes have brought the incidence of complications after intubation of children to negligible proportions no greater than that in adults.

Intubation of neonates and infants of one month or less is particularly hazardous and should consequently be carried out only by an experienced anaesthetist. The anterior tilting of the larynx makes it sometimes difficult to see and it is easy for the laryngoscope blade to overshoot the epiglottis and place the tube in the oesophagus. Gentle pressure backwards by an assistant during laryngoscopy is helpful to avoid this hazard. Should technical difficulties of this sort be encountered following induction of apnoea by relaxant, maintenance of adequate ventilation could prove very difficult. The placing of an endotracheal tube in the oesophagus is a hazard at any age. It should be remembered that when pre-oxygenation takes place, or a child is induced with oxygen and an inhalational agent, a tube in the oesophagus may not be immediately followed by cyanosis, which may not appear until 2-3 min has elapsed. Therefore, every effort should be made to confirm that the tube is in the trachea after intubation of infants by auscultation of the chest.

Control of the airway of a paralysed child even in the higher age groups can be difficult and those unfamiliar with intubating children should make their first attempts under inhalational anaesthesia when the child is responsible for its own respiration. Later, when the anaesthetist is familiar with viewing infantile larynxes, attempts using relaxants can be made.

### 36.6.1  Anatomical Considerations

Before attempting intubation of infants, attention must be given to the differences between the infantile larynx and that of the mature adult.

1) In infants the larynx is higher than in adults and opposite the fourth cervical instead of the seventh cervical vertebra.

2) In infants the epiglottis is curved like an inverted V, instead of being flat as in an adult.

3) The narrowest part of the infantile larynx is at the level of the

cricoid cartilage and not at the vocal cords as in adults, and the direction of its long axis is forwards and downwards, not downwards alone as in the adult.

### 36.6.2  Technical Considerations

For the above reasons a straight-blade laryngoscope placed posterior to the epiglottis is preferable to the curved Mackintosh blade which goes anteriorly and does not flatten the inverted V shape epiglottis of the infant, making it necessary to depress the larynx with a finger in order to bring it into view.

*Choice.* For neonates a 3.5 tube is suitable for all except those under 2 kg in weight, when a number 3 tube is satisfactory. Errors in judgement in choice of tubes are inevitable and a size larger or smaller than that selected should always be put out in case they are necessary.

Secure metal connectors between the tube and the tubing of the Ayre's T-piece are very important and should always be tested before induction begins. Nothing is worse after successful intubation than to find the endotracheal connector slipping off the endotracheal tube, or that one is unable to fit the other end onto the connected tubing of the Ayre's T-piece.

### 36.7  Muscle Relaxation

It is easy to obtain satisfactory muscular relaxation in children with inhalational agents. Control of respiration is quite easy with halothane, owing to its non-irritant properties.

When using muscle relaxants for children care is necessary to calculate the correct dosage. Neonates are said to be more sensitive to tubocurarine until three or four weeks of age. The dose of tubocurarine recommended is 0.51 mg followed by 0.25 mg except in the case of neonates when 0.15 mg presuambly would be sufficient. Suxamethonium is satisfactory in twice the weight equivalent dose for adults, that is to say 5 mg repeated as needed.

Reversal of non-depolarising relaxants is by means of neostigmine in a dose of 1 mg and atropine 0.3 mg rising to 0.6 mg in children over 1 year of age.

### 36.8  Monitoring Pulse and Respiration

In order to have a continuous audible record of pulse and respiration, many anaesthetists use a precordial stethoscope taped to the chest wall and connected to an ear piece. Alternatively, oesophageal inflatable scopes are available also with an ear piece. Some cotton wool over the end of the expiratory arm of the Ayre's T-piece is also a help at ensuring respiration is continuing adequately. It is vital to have some means of checking that the breathing is adequate in depth and not obstructed.

## 36.9 Estimating Blood Loss

Neonate blood volume is about 350 ml, hence accurate record of blood loss is absolutely essential in major surgery. Swab weighing itself is not sufficiently accurate. The best method is to extract the haemoglobin from all swabs and linen in a known volume of water and estimate the haemoglobin concentration resulting by conventional means.

## 36.10 Intravenous Electrolytes

Ringer lactate 2 ml/kg is recommended as a standard intravenous therapy for neonates and infants. Use of normal saline carries a danger of oedema from sodium excess.

## 36.11 Temperature Changes During Anaesthesia

Neonates and infants lose heat easily and this loss is accelerated by failure to humidify and warm anaesthetic gases, particularly during thoracotomies and laparotomies. Most units have heated blankets thermostatically controlled on the operating table. However, during thoracotomies and laparotomies, some means of heating and raising the humidity of anaesthetic gases by passage over warm water is recommended. During control of respiration as already mentioned the to and fro Waters type absorber offers a very convenient way of conserving heat and moisture. Constant postoperative supervision is vital and facilities for mechanical assistance of respiration must always be available.

# 37 Dental Surgery

Most dental anaesthesia is carried out either in the dentist's surgery or in the outpatient department of a clinic. The hazards of day surgery set out in Chap. 46 apply to all these patients who should receive the same instructions about preparation and conditions of returning home. The anaesthetic technique must ensure rapid recovery.

## 37.1 Assessment

Dental patients being ambulant have no obvious disabling cardiac or respiratory handicap but should a history of either be obtained, local analgesia should be advised, otherwise general anaesthesia as an in-patient. Some patients, although healthy are difficult to anaesthetise in a dental surgery and anaesthetists should learn to anticipate trouble.

Nervous, highly strung adults, or excitable, imaginative children between the ages of 7 and 15 years are often unwilling to submit to inhalational or intravenous induction. Pre-operative sedation is sometimes helpful, for adults, a grain of phenobarbitone or 10 g diazepam a couple of hours before the procedure and for children, trimeprazine or promethazine in a dose appropriate for their weight and age.

Athletes, muscular labourers and alcoholics are impossible to anaesthetise with nitrous oxide alone. Whenever possible it is better to avoid general anaesthesia in a dental surgery and if local analgesia is not practicable, advise full general anaesthetic in a properly equipped clinic.

Physically and mentally handicapped children often need prolonged conservative dentistry, with nasotracheal anaesthesia. They are not suitable subjects for beginners.

## 37.2  Anaesthetic Techniques in the Dental Chair

### 37.2.1  Upright or Horizontal?

There is controversy about the safety of anaesthetising patients in a sitting position because fainting due to fall in blood pressure could cause cardiac arrest and brain damage. A fainting attack is usually preceded by a period of immobility and a partial deafferentation of the central nervous system associated with preponderance of vagal tone and sympathetic depression. Dental patients about to undergo general anaesthesia are usually alert, often apprehensive, with increased circulating catecholamines sufficient to offset any vagal inhibitory processes. During induction they are either actively engaged in breathing a gas, or in squeezing their hands to bring out veins for intravenous injection and steeling themselves to remain immobile against the pain of the needle. The fainting theory must be regarded as 'not proven'. It is well known, however, that any intravenous induction is accompanied by a fall in blood pressure, as is even the passage from wakefulness to sleep. In modern dental practice a compromise has actually been reached, since most dental chairs accommodate patients in a semi-reclining position acceptable to those who agree with the fainting theories.

### 37.2.2  Induction and Maintenance

In the dental chair, induction and maintenance of anaesthesia are achieved either by an inhalational technique with nitrous oxide and oxygen supplemented by a volatile agent, or by an intravenous induction and maintenance by nitrous oxide oxygen and volatile agents, or by supplementary intravenous agents through an indwelling needle.

### 37.2.3  Particular Hazards

Although the hazards of any anaesthetic apply to dental anaesthesia, there are certain particular risks that arise because two people are competing for access to the airway, while the position of the anaesthetist behind the patient and that of the dental surgeon in front restrict direct observation of the patient's respiration.

*Airway Obstruction.* Stertorous respiration is a sign of an obstructed airway. Usually it can be overcome by pulling the patient's jaw forward or by use of a nasopharyngeal tube. The latter, however, can cause nasal bleeding and is best avoided by the inexperienced.

Obstruction developing during extraction and conservation work can easily arise from a displaced pack. Surprisingly it often escapes notice until cyanosis appears (indicating at least one third of the available haemoglobin is in a reduced state) and cardiac arrest is imminent. This is not always due to carelessness because observation of fully clothed dental patients is more difficult than of patients half-naked on an operating table.

During partial or even complete respiratory obstruction, abdominal movement continues, but retraction of the ribs (a diagnostic sign) is not always obvious in fully clothed patients. Absence of effective chest movement should draw the anaesthetist's attention to defective respiration but this also is not so obvious because the anaesthetist stands behind and the dental surgeon in front of the patient, partially or even totally obscuring the thorax from view. These are reasons why anaesthetists should be even more vigilant than usual with patients in a dental chair, especially if the procedure lasts longer than a few minutes. Indeed, during long conservation, unless an airway is ensured by means of an endotracheal tube, there is much to be said for a pause every five minutes.

Clinical measurements taken on patients undergoing conservative procedures under intermittent intravenous anaesthesia by an experienced anaesthetist have shown an unacceptably high incidence of partial respiratory obstruction, arterial hypoxaemia, tachycardia and fall in peripheral resistance. These findings have been challenged, but demonstration of the existence of partial respiratory obstruction and arterial hypoxaemia in experienced hands is good reason why those without experience should avoid similar techniques.

### 37.2.4  Cardiovascular Complications

A fall in systolic blood pressure sometimes accompanies intravenous induction and for this reason the patient should always be in a reclining position. This has been discussed already. Pressure on the carotid sinus during support of the jaw could cause bradycardia.

Pressure on the internal carotid arteries of each side during support of the lower jaw for difficult root extractions could also cause complications. There are on record two cases of death after dental anaesthesia administered by an established consultant, in which postmortem examination showed cerebral softening in areas supplied by the middle and posterior cerebral arteries, although areas of distribution of the vertebral vessels were unaffected. Such changes could be the result of occlusion of the carotid arteries above the point of origin of the vertebral arteries; this would not interfere with the blood supply of pons and medulla, explaining why no changes in breathing or cardiovascular reflexes occurred.

### 37.2.5  Respiratory Complications

Respiratory complications are commoner following intravenous agents than inhalational methods. Treatment is more difficult because of the time it takes for intravenous agents to be metabolised.

Stridor and spasm may occur from the presence of phlegm or inhaled blood on the larynx or from strong sensory stimulation. Discontinuation of an inhalational agent allows rapid recovery, but recovery is longer after an intravenous induction, and oxygen should be given, with a face mask and light pressure on the reservoir bag, to prevent oxygen lack during return of normal respiration.

Cessation of respiration may arise from breath-holding, deep anaesthesia or oxygen lack. Breath-holding usually occurs during inhalational induction; the mask or nose-piece should be left in place, whilst rising blood level of carbon dioxide stimulates respiration and increases depth of anaesthesia.

Anaesthesia of sufficient depth to cause respiratory failure should never occur during dental anaesthesia. Although oxygenation will initially appear satisfactory, unless the administration is stopped immediately and the lungs inflated with air or oxygen, cardiac arrest from oxygen lack can easily follow. Respiratory failure from oxygen lack is a desperate situation. It is accompanied by dilated pupils, grey cyanotic skin, mucous membranes and finger nails, and a failing or absent pulse.

The patient should be taken from the chair and placed on the floor and after excluding respiratory obstruction from a displaced pack clearing the airway, inflation of the lungs should start either with mouth to mouth breathing or with oxygen, whilst an assistant performs cardiac massage. If an empty oxygen cylinder is the cause, mouth to mouth respiration should continue until another one is found. If the heart does not begin to beat, cardiac massage should be continued and the procedure for cardiac arrest (see Chap. 23) carried out.

## 37.3 In-patients

Whilst most dental procedures can be undertaken in the dental chair, treatment as an in-patient is preferred:

1) When postoperative pain, discomfort, swelling or infection could follow, for example after removal of impacted wisdom teeth.

2) When the poor physical condition of the patient contra-indicates anaesthesia in the dental chair. Examples are mentally defective children, spastics and those with known cardiac disease, haemorrhagic disorders, haemophilia or sickling trait.

3) For extensive periodontal procedures lasting over 1 h.

The anaesthetic technique involved includes passage of an endotracheal tube through the nose and insertion of a throat pack, according to the dental surgeon's requirements. All throat packs have a tape attached which lies outside the mouth after insertion and to which a metal clip should be always attached to ensure its removal afterwards. Fatal respiratory obstruction has been recorded from a 'forgotten' pack.

At the end of the operation the nasal tube should remain in place after removal of the pack until the pharynx has been cleared of blood and debris and the patient placed in the lateral position with the head low. The tube can be removed when the patient is able to cough after insertion of an oral airway.

# 38 Ophthalmic Surgery

Two main hazards during anaesthesia for ophthalmic surgery are the oculocardiac reflex, and vitreous loss during intra-ocular procedures. Hazards during recovery include vomiting, coughing and restlessness.

## 38.1  Oculocardiac Reflex

Stimuli from several parts of the eye can cause cardiac arrhythmias, but the most sensitive are the ocular muscles. Traction on muscles or other stimuli induce reflex vagal activity. This becomes evident as bradycardia, which may be followed by cardiac arrest.

Atropine premedication and gallamine used as relaxants are helpful preventive measures because they reduce vagal tone, but the best of all is adequate depth of anaesthesia, especially during squint operations on young children. A suitable technique would include light premedication including atropine, intravenous induction with gallamine for relaxation before intubation in older children and inhalational anaesthesia for younger children. Anaesthetists must ensure that the first plane of the third stage of anaesthesia is established before allowing traction on the ophthalmic muscles. Some authorities recommend a continuous ECG or pulse monitoring. A finger on the pulse quickly detects bradycardia and is free from mechanical fault.

## 38.2  Intra-ocular Surgery

Some years ago, local anaesthetic was widely used for intra-ocular surgery because procedures were short. The introduction of operating microscopes and the availability of very fine sutures has slowed up the surgical pace and lengthened the procedures, so that general anaesthesia has replaced local analgesia. Difficulties in maintaining a clear airway during these longer procedures has led to adoption of endotracheal anaesthesia, previously unpopular because occasional bouts of coughing increased intra-ocular tension and added to operative difficulties. Use of suture material has reduced the harm from such complications during recovery.

Anaesthesia for intra-ocular surgery should not cause increase of intra-ocular tension, should avoid coughing and spasm during induction and maintenance, and provide calm recovery without restlessness, coughing or vomiting.

### 38.2.1  Intra-ocular Tension

*Increase* of intra-ocular tension occurs:

1) Following injection of depolarising relaxants like suxamethonium. The effect is temporary and returns to normal with return of muscle movement, i.e. within 3-5 min. If the patient receives a second injection, the pressure will rise again, and if the eye is 'open', vitreous prolapse may occur.

2) During oxygen lack, carbon dioxide accumulation and coughing.

3) With gross rises in arterial central venous pressure.

*Reduction* of intra-ocular tension is associated with:

1) Hyperventilation and the accompanying reduction of the blood carbon dioxide.

2) Administration of volatile anaesthetic agents, particularly halothane.

3) Administration of narcotic agents.

4) Administration of phenothiazines, particularly chlorpromazine, given as part of the premedication, or intravenously as part of the anaesthetic technique.

5) Reduction of arterial blood pressure to around 11 kPa. Small increases in arterial blood pressure or central venous pressure do not have any material effect.

### 38.2.2  Anaesthetic Technique

*Premedication.* A calm, nausea-free recovery is most likely to result from inclusion of phenothiazine derivatives with pethidine as premedication. Chlorpromazine has all the qualities required during and after operation; it lowers the intra-ocular pressure and reduces the incidence of post-operative vomiting. Heavy opiate dosage is unnecessary because due to absence of pain recovery is delayed.

*Induction.* Although in theory suxamethonium is contra-indicated because it raises intra-ocular pressure, many anaesthetists use it as its effects have worn off during the 5 min elapsing between induction and the beginning of surgery. Non-depolarising relaxants are preferable. Their longer action allows full control of respiration with 1% halothane to be established before the effects of the relaxant have worn off. Generous spraying of the trachea and vocal cords with 4% lignocaine helps reduce tracheal irritability. Most patients for cataract surgery are elderly and do not require large doses of anaesthetics, although occasional patients from younger age groups (possibly heavy smokers) will require larger amounts. Failure to make this allowance increases the risk of coughing and straining on the tube, which in presence of an open eye raises intra-ocular tension and causes loss of vitreous.

*Recovery.* Recovery after ophthalmic surgery is slow, since painful stimulus from the operating area is not very great. Provided the pharynx is clear, the tube can be removed and an airway inserted before active coughing occurs. When this is done, the head should be kept low, and the patient turned into the lateral position. With modern sutures no harm results from delaying extubation until a response to its presence is evident.

## 38.3 Emergency Ophthalmic Surgery

The need for ophthalmic emergency surgery arises from traumatic conditions, including penetrating injuries of the eye, for complications of cataract extraction (prolapse of the iris), and lens extraction as a last resort in acute glaucoma. A rise in intra-ocular pressure must be avoided in all cases and the precautions already outlined should be observed.

Procedures are not usually prolonged, and intravenous induction followed by nitrous oxide, oxygen and halothane with an oral airway, protects against rise in intra-ocular pressure due to cough and straining on an endotracheal tube during maintenance or recovery.

It is not difficult to control a patient with an oral airway during ophthalmic surgery. Metal airway caps are available which slide over the metal flange of a Guedel airway, and the Matthias airway has a cap permanently attached. If intubation is undertaken, suxamethonium should not be used, as the eye is already open or under tension.

During recovery, pain may cause contraction of the orbicularis muscle, resulting in a rise of intra-ocular pressure. This can be prevented by a local block of the facial nerve as it crosses the neck of the mandible (4 ml of 0.5% bupivacaine in 1:200 000 adrenaline) at the end of the operation.

# 39 Burns

## 39.1 Classification

Burns are classified according to the depth of injury. First degree consists only of loss of epidermis and is followed by healing within a few days. With the second degree, although there is partial loss of dermis, sufficient epithelial tissue remains to allow resurfacing to occur. These two types of burn are therefore much less serious and dangerous than the third degree burn in which there is full thickness loss of skin, all the epithelial elements are destroyed and the only way of covering the raw area is by skin grafting after removal of the burnt eschar. An extensive burn is defined as one which involves 18% or more of the body surface of an adult (the entire chest and abdomen or the entire back) or more than 12% in a child under 12 years of age. Figure 4 illustrates a rough and ready method for estimating percentage of body surface burnt.

## 39.2 Care of Patients Before Operation

Burnt patients loose fluids rapidly. Capillary permeability increases and dilation and rupture of small vessels in the burnt area account for the greater part of the fluid loss, which continues for 48 h or more after the burn. Blood loss is not great unless the burn is really deep but the red blood corpuscles become more fragile and as haematopoiesis is depressed anaemia is common.

Before any active treatment of the burn can take place, treatment of hypovolaemic shock by intravenous infusion of fresh frozen plasma or dextran 100 should be started. The quantity needed varies with the extent of the burn.

Anaesthesia is not usually required for burnt patients in the early stages but is needed after about 14 days, when eschar over the burn area is ready for removal and replacement by skin grafts. At this stage the

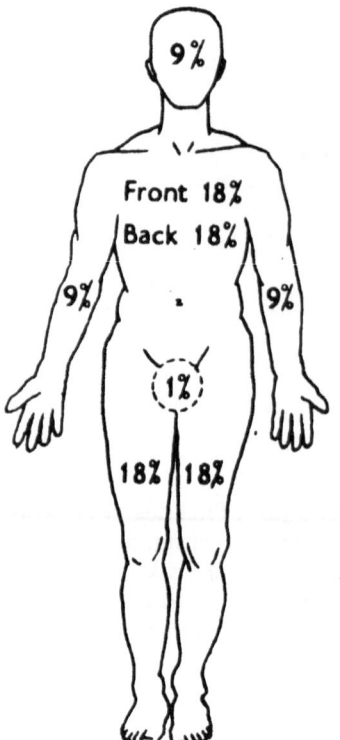

**Fig. 4.** 'Rule of nines' for estimating the percentage of body surface burned. From Thornton HL, Norton-Perkins HD (1974) Emergency anaesthesia, 2nd edn. Arnold, London. Copyright 1974, American Medical Association.

condition of the patient depends on the extent and degree of infection and associated toxaemia. Anaemia is always present. Daily haemoglobin estimates are made as a routine and patients receive transfusion when the haemoglobin levels fall too low. Transfusions and high protein diet are the best measures to ensure optimum physical state before anaesthesia. In spite of this treatment some patients do deteriorate, but every effort must be made to anaesthetise them since their only chance of survival is removal of the sloughs and skin grafting.

## 39.3 Premedication

Since burnt patients appear to be prone to cardiac arrest, premedication should aim at reducing circulating catecholamines by prescribing drugs to relieve anxiety and tension as well as suppression of autonomic reflex activity. Phenothiazines are particularly suitable, either promethazine or chlorpromazine. An opiate analgesic should be included to suppress the intense pain these patients experience during recovery.

## 39.4  Hazards During Anaesthesia

There are three main dangers in anaesthesia for the treatment of burns:

1) Too little anaesthetic increases the risk of cardiac arrest from increased autonomic reflex activity, to which burnt patients are particularly susceptible. Anaesthetists with experience of treatment of burns recommend not less than 1 % halothane for maintenance.

2) Lack of oxygen must be avoided. Kidney, lung and liver may all have already been damaged by anoxia during the shock phase and are therefore more than usually susceptible to further deprivation.

3) Blood loss replacement during removal of the eschar should be rapid and accurate. Anaesthetists should appreciate the possibility of brisk bleeding during removal of sloughs, especially if two or three surgeons (as often happens) work together. Replacement must be rapid, if necessary under pressure, and the surgeons can be asked to pause and control haemorrhage with pressure if replacement appears to fall behind blood loss. Intravenous therapy itself in burnt patients presents problems because good veins are often difficult to find.

## 39.5  Children

Rectal thiopentone for young children has many supporters, but as pain causes restlessness under barbiturate sedation, an intravenous injection of an opiate prior to recovery is always necessary. As already mentioned, anaesthesia shold be of sufficient depth to prevent any reflex activity affecting the heart, but should not be so deep as to delay recovery and the early resumption of a high protein diet. Induction by a short-acting barbiturate such as methohexitone and maintenance with halothane, nitrous oxide and oxygen is a common routine. Repeated anaesthesia is unavoidable and although children in burn units receive repeated halothane administrations, jaundice is conspicuous by its absence.

Endotracheal intubation is necessary for treatment of burns of face, head and neck. Some avoid the use of suxamethonium for fear of increasing the risk of cardiac arrest, as some burnt patients have a high blood calcium which suxamethonium further increases. On the other hand, intubation under too light a plane of anaesthesia can also predispose to cardiac irregularities of reflex origin.

With the recently introduced anaesthetic agent ketamine, effective by intravenous and intramuscular routes, the swallowing reflex is not abolished. Gastric reflux therefore presents no problem and restriction of diet before anaesthesia is not necessary, and rapid recovery allows early resumption of full diet. This is a great advantage in the maintenance of nutrition, so essential to successful treatment.

For this reason ketamine has become popular for children who need repeated painful dressings. It must be remembered, however, that recovery should be undisturbed and take place in a quiet area because emotional disturbance does occur, especially in slightly older children. This is the only reason why ketamine has not become more popular.

# 40 Thoracic Surgery

Development of surgery within the thoracic cavity was delayed for years because of the dangers which arise from opening the chest in anaesthetised patients. When this occurs in a patient who is breathing spontaneously, the subatmospheric pressure on the opened side rises to equal that of the atmosphere and the lung collapses due to the recoil of its elastic fibres. There thus arises a difference in pressure between the opened side and the closed side, so that the mediastinum and its contents, the heart and blood vessels, are drawn over to the sound side. In the absence of treatment the ensuing respiratory and cardiovascular disturbances can lead to death in a short time.

## 40.1 Respiratory Disturbances

When the chest is opened, paradoxical respiration occurs. During inspiration the lung on the sound side draws air from the lung on the affected side and on expiration passes this air back into the affected lung. Thus the affected lung expands during expiration and contracts during inspiration, so interfering with gaseous exchange.

The carbon dioxide content of the air in the affected lung increases progressively as it passes back and forth between the two lungs. This is at the expense of oxygenation, so that $PaO_2$ falls progressively in spite of the stimulation of breathing from the raised carbon dioxide, whose only effect is intensification of the circulatory disturbances.

## 40.2 Circulatory Disturbances

The absence of subatmospheric pressure in the chest, which normally draws blood into the right side of the heart, means that venous return and cardiac output fall.

The movement of the mediastinum towards the sound side on inspiration and back again on expiration causes intermittent obstruction of the superior and inferior vena cava and sets up reflex induced tachycardia and low blood pressure. This movement is reduced in the presence of old inflammatory disease in the mediastinum which has produced fibrous changes. The cardiovascular changes can be reduced by infiltrating the pulmonary plexus at the hilum of the lung or vagus nerve in the back. The end result of this mediastinal movement is a clinical picture of shock arising from reflex disturbances of autonomic origin.

## 40.3  Control of an Open Chest

The above-mentioned complications arising from opening the chest can be controlled by artificial respiration which requires some way of abolishing respiratory movement. Before relaxants became available this was achieved by exploiting the respiratory depressant action of cyclopropane and reduction of respiratory drive by absorbing carbon dioxide in soda lime after manual ventilation. Dr. Nosworthy in the U.K. and Dr. Guedel in the U.S.A. pioneered this method in 1940 and 1941 and made intrathoracic operations possible for the first time. This technique came ultimately to be known as 'controlled respiration'.

After introduction of relaxants it became possible to control breathing by paralysis of the muscles of respiration. A technique of muscular paralysis with light general anaesthesia is now standard for intrathoracic procedures. A more recent method which involves central depression of the respiratory centre to the point of apnoea with potent opiates like fentanyl is known as neuroleptanalgesia. Supplementary nitrous oxide is essential to ensure unconsciousness. Delayed respiratory depression after fentanyl in large doses from a poorly understood cumulative effect suggests that this method should be avoided by those who do not have experience of the method in other fields.

## 40.4  Pulmonary Secretions

Control of pulmonary secretions was a much greater problem in the early days of thoracic surgery before antibiotics and chemotherapy had reduced the incidence and severity of tuberculosis and bronchiectasis. Nevertheless, they do pose a serious problem and demand attention in any of the following conditions:

1) Bronchiectasis
2) Empyema and broncho-pleural fistula
3) Lung abscesses
4) Carcinoma of the bronchus
5) Haemorrhage from adenoma

6) Tuberculous cavities

7) Haemorrhage following biopsy of a bronchus

There are various methods of dealing with secretions.

Preoperatively, postural drainage supervised by an experienced physio-therapist and antiobiotic therapy can reduce secretions, especially in chronic inflammatory conditions like bronchiectasis.

The use of regional analgesia for conditions like empyema and thoracoplasty for tuberculosis can, under paravertebral block, allow retention of the cough reflex so that patients control their own secretions.

Posture combined with intermittent suction during operation after adoption of a head-down tilt allows secretions to enter the endotracheal tube and be removed by suction. To do this satisfactorily certain conditions must be met. If the patient is in the lateral position, a tilt of 40°-50° is needed to avoid secretions from the upper lung passing into the healthy side. When the left lung is uppermost, a tilt of 30° is satisfactory, but when the right lung is uppermost, it must be 40° or more. Such a degree of tilt makes surgical approach difficult and most surgeons now prefer to have the patient prone with a head-down tilt.

The most popular method is that described by Parry Brown (Fig. 5). The patient is placed in the prone position so that the affected lung is uppermost allowing continuous free drainage into the trachea. A well filled pillow is placed under the pelvis and a padded block under the chest reaching as far as the manubrium sterni. The operated side should hang slightly over the table with the arm hanging downwards. This allows a larger incision and draws the scapula away from the operative field.

The head should be extended at the occipito-atlanteal joint and turned to the side of the operation to prevent kinking of the contralateral main bronchus during traction on the hilum. This position ensures a stable mediastinum, is suitable for children, and prevents spillage into the

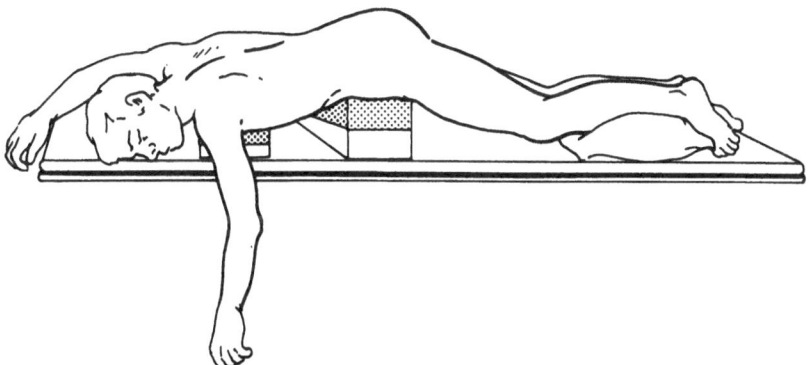

**Fig. 5.** Prone position (Parry Brown) for drainage of secretions. Adapted from Churchill-Davidson HC (1978) A practice of anaesthesia, 4th edn. Lloyd-Luke (Medical Books), London.

healthy lung. Disadvantages are limitation of exposure for the surgeon and difficulty in access to the endotracheal tube by the anaesthetist. Kinking of the tube can be prevented using a new nylon-reinforced flexible tube.

Other devices for control of secretions include bronchial blockers, double lumen tubes (Robertshaw and Carlen), and one lung anaesthesia. Their employment is not recommended to those who have not had training in their use. The majority of lung resections can be carried out safely and satisfactorily with an endotracheal tube, controlled respiration and intermittent suction. It must be remembered that over-enthusiastic and prolonged suction causes serious oxygen lack.

### 40.5  Other Problems

All patients should have an intravenous drip, but blood loss is not usually great except in decortication operations.

Deflation of the lung on the operated side can be assisted by reducing the inflation pressure when the chest is opened and even allowing a few minutes' apnoea.

Suture of the bronchus following resection with a clamp in place presents no difficulty. Sometimes a clamp is not used and in these circumstances the anaesthetist should insist on vigorous hyperventilation with oxygen before it is cut. Usually no difficulties are encountered during the procedure. Should delay lead to cyanosis of the patient, the surgeon can be asked to plug the hole with a gauze swab to allow oxygenation.

At the end of the operation during closure of the wound anaesthetists should inflate the lungs vigorously to expel as much air from the chest as possible. The remaining air is usually removed through a drainage tube connected to an underwater seal.

# 41 Vascular Surgery

The extent and scope of peripheral vascular surgery has increased in recent years. In the main, it is confined to the abdominal aorta and lower limbs and occasionally to internal carotid arteries.

## 41.1  Assessment

The presence of arterial disease is seldom if ever confined to one blood vessel and extensive vascular disease elsewhere especially of the coronary artery must be assumed to be present. Pre-operative ECGs and cardiac assessment are therefore essential preliminaries to anaesthesia.

## 41.2  Operations Confined to Lower Limb

Femoro-popliteal bypass with a vein graft or prosthesis is a straight-forward procedure not requiring any special technique and intubation is optional. A good intravenous line must always be set up and infusion of electrolytes or blood should be on the generous side. Heparin is always used and the need to reverse it after operation should be remembered.

Conventional techniques depend mainly on the nitrous oxide, oxygen and relaxant sequence supplemented by intravenous pethidine, neurolept-analgesic drugs (combination of droperidol and fentanyl), or by small doses of halothane or other inhalational agents. This technique maintains a high level of blood pressure throughout the procedure.

## 41.3  Major Arterial Surgery

### 41.3.1  Replacement of Abdominal Aorta

Maintenance of systolic blood pressure is the prior interest of the surgeon whatever technique is used, combined with adequate perfusion of the extremities. Some vasodilatation from epidurals, halothane or chlorpromazine is tolerated provided generous intravenous infusion compensates for the accompanying 25% increase in capacitance of the vascular bed.

Vasodilator techniques by induction of epidural analgesia or use of intravenous chlorpromazine and pethidine with relaxant and nitrous oxide and oxygen with minimal halothane provide good operating conditions and reduce blood loss. Recovery is slow but blood pressure rises progressively and the sudden fall that often accompanies an injection of Omnopon for relief of pain after rapid recovery does not occur. There is no doubt that patients who receive epidurals or chlorpromazine have a reduced incidence of postoperative ileus which is a most distressing complication to the patient.

Large-bore cannulae should be used for intravenous lines so that rapid replacement of fluids can take place when necessary. Central venous pressure lines are used as a routine measure in many units to assist in estimation of intravenous fluid requirements, especially in the post-operative phase.

The most hazardous moment of abdominal aortic replacement occurs when the graft has been put in place and the clamp is taken off the abdominal aorta. This is always followed by a significant fall in blood pressure which can, to some extent, be reduced by keeping the isolated part of the circulation well filled. Dilated veins help to accommodate the extra fluid.

Although the lower limbs may be deprived of circulation for up to an hour during the placing in position of the graft, metabolic acidosis which would be expected does not occur to any significant degree.

### 41.3.2 Leaking Aortic Aneurysm

Emergency anaesthesia for surgery to replace a leaking abdominal aortic aneurysm is one of the most hazardous procedures in surgery and carries a mortality in the region of 50%.

Patients invariably present in a state of shock with cyanosed extremities, sweating and palor. Vein spasm is frequently so intense that it is almost impossible to set up an intravenous drip and even when it is set up to get the fluid into the veins.

In such circumstances the author has found that small intravenous doses of 5 mg chlorpromazine (diluted 50 mg in 20 ml saline) help to dilate the peripheral circulation and allow more rapid infusion of much-needed fluid. Alternatively or simultaneously inhalation of 0.5% halothane in oxygen improves perfusion. Once the drips are running freely, rapid infusion of blood or fresh frozen plasma or electrolytes under pressure should continue until systolic blood pressure is in the region of 11-12 kPa and peripheral perfusion adequate, at which moment the operation may start.

The value of chlorpromazine in haemorrhagic shock should cause no surprise since it reduces the secretion of anti-diuretic hormone (pitressin) following pain and haemorrhage which is known to play a leading part in development of haemorrhagic shock (see also Chap. 26).

The hazards of massive transfusion (see Sect. 21.2) are particularly relevant since patients require large quantities (20-25 units) of blood during the operation. A warming device must always be included in the intravenous set-up in order to avoid accidental hypothermia. The presence of shock at the beginning of the procedure makes the likelihood of metabolic acidosis in this condition more likely than in the planned procedure described above. An intravenous infusion of 8.4% sodium bicarbonate will help to correct this.

### 41.3.3  Carotid Endarterectomy

Arterial disease of the carotid artery can lead to cerebral ischaemia of sufficient content to cause personality change, loss of memory and increased sensitivity to central nervous depressant drugs.

Clamping of the internal carotid during attempts to clear the carotid artery could reduce the already difficult circulation and cause permanent cerebral damage.

In practice cerebral damage does not always occur because a reasonably good collateral circulation has already been established. The study of arteriograms before operation is often very helpful in establishing this. Anaesthetic techniques ensure optimum brain perfusion by avoidance of hypotensive episodes and of vasoconstriction. Reflex bradycardia may occur from manipulation near the carotid sinus but this can be prevented by previous infiltration of local analgesic or the administration of intravenous atropine. Surface cooling of patients to 30° has been advocated as a suitable technique.

# 42 Miscellaneous Surgical Procedures

## 42.1  Phaeochromocytoma

Phaeochromocytoma is a tumour of chromaffin cells of the adrenal medulla which secretes adrenaline and noradrenaline with resulting hypertension.

It is not confined to the adrenal gland and can be found near the aortic bifurcation, in the coeliac plexus, in the paravertebral spaces and even the appendix. Patients present with persistent high blood pressure or paroxysms of hypertension.

Before a decision for surgery, blood pressure has been brought under control by phenoxybenzamine (Dibenyline) or phentolamine. Blood volume is sometimes reduced and if this is the case, pre-operative correction is advisable by very slow transfusion to avoid precipitating a paroxysm of hypertension.

### 42.1.1  Premedication
Chlorpromazine has been recommended together with pethidine to ensure a well sedated patient before operation. As, however, it has only a slight peripheral anti-adrenal action it does not protect against increase of circulatory noradrenaline following stimuli.

### 42.1.2  Anaesthetic Technique
Smooth, tranquil conditions must be provided, without coughing and spasm.

Induction with thiopentone followed by intubation under a long acting relaxant with nitrous oxide, oxygen and halothane for maintenance with controlled respiration provides good operating conditions. The surgical approach is usually retroperitoneal with the patient in the prone or lateral position. The possibility of accidental pneumothorax must always be borne in mind.

During operation constant blood pressure measurements are essential. Halothane helps to control hypertensive responses to surgery but figures exceeding 33 kPa indicate the need for control with phentolamine (Rogitine) 5 mg intravenously. Sodium nitroprusside has also been recommended as a means of controlling hypertensive spasms during operation. Following removal of the tumour low blood pressure may give rise to concern and some authorities recommend a noradrenaline drip 4 mg/l or phenylephrine 20 mg/l during the postoperative period. In many centres these measures are no longer thought necessary. Systolic pressures between 9.3 and 10.7 kPa are accepted and are not an indication for vasopressor solutions.

## 42.2 Thyroidectomy

In bygone days the circulatory complications of thyrotoxicosis presented a major hazard for anaesthesia but after preparation with thiouracil and Lugol's iodine, patients requiring anaesthesia today have a stable cardio-vascular system, controlled atrial fibrillation being the commonest abnormality. In patients with large glands, some deviation of the trachea may be present. Prolongation of the tumour behind the sternum is another cause of deviation. Problems of intubation may therefore be experienced. All patients should have pre-anaesthetic X-ray of the neck and upper thorax so that any such abnormalities can be clearly defined.

### 42.2.1 Premedication
Sedative premedication benefits patients for thyroid surgery since they are often nervous whilst a slow and peaceful recovery reduces complications (see Sect. 42.2.5).

### 42.2.2 Anaesthetic Technique
The aim of anaesthesia is to keep congestion of the neck veins to a minimum and prevent coughing and spasm during the surgical manipulations required to deliver the enlarged lobes.

In the past some surgeons preferred not to have their patients intubated in order to reduce postoperative tracheitis but intubation is essential if X-rays show deviation or compression of the trachea, the presence of a retrosternal goitre or if malignancy is suspected.

Few present-day anaesthetists would undertake anaesthesia for this condition without the passage of an endotracheal tube. However, until a few years ago instrument catalogues contained an illustration of a flattened face mask designed for use during thyroidectomy.

The author's technique consists of premedication with 50 mg chlorpromazine and pethidine followed by the same quantities dissolved in 20 ml saline given intravenously as induction followed by 150-200 mg thiopentone, 100 mg suxamethonium and passage of a nylon-reinforced flexible endotracheal tube. Anaesthesia continues with 1-2% halothane with a modest foot-down tilt. Respiration is spontaneous throughout.

The advantages are minimal congestion of the neck veins, no coughing or straining on delivery of the gland and slow recovery without nausea and vomiting. Nausea and vomiting is a commoner postoperative complication of thyroid surgery than is realised. Disturbance of the vagal nerves in the neck may be a reason.

Conventional techniques with relaxant, nitrous oxide, oxygen, halothane and intubation preceded by generous laryngo-tracheal local analgesic spray also provide acceptable operating conditions.

### 42.2.3  Infiltration

Many surgeons infiltrate the subcutaneous tissues over the thyroid gland with 1:200 000 adrenaline in saline to produce vasoconstriction and reduce bleeding. This activity is often delegated to the anaesthetist so that more time can elapse between infiltration and incision, ensuring better vasoconstriction. (See however comments on this practice in Chaps. 17 and 30; modern anaesthesia surely makes it superfluous.)

### 42.2.4  Postoperative care

At the end of the operation removal of the tube can take place before active return of the cough reflex but should be preceded by gentle suction (see, however, Chap. 38). Excessive coughing and straining after thyroid operations can cause postoperative oozing, haemorrhage and haematoma formation. After extubation the surgeon may ask the anaesthetist to examine the vocal cords to ensure that movement is full and normal and no damage to the recurrent laryngeal nerve has occurred. Sometimes laryngoscopy for this purpose is also undertaken prior to intubation.

### 42.2.5  Recovery

During recovery several complications can occur.

Reactionary haemorrhage (usually after coughing) may cause partial obstruction and require emergency aspiration and further anaesthesia to re-open the wound and stop the bleeding.

Oedema of the larynx has been described on the second or third postoperative day. Stridor will suggest the diagnosis which is confirmed by indirect laryngoscopy. If it increases, tracheostomy may be necessary.

Injury to the recurrent laryngeal nerve may occur. It may be transient or permanent. Unilateral lesions cause little trouble except to singers, actors or others who use their voice professionally. A bilateral permanent paralysis can cause sufficient airway obstruction to require tracheostomy.

Collapse of the trachea, often described, is a rare complication unless cartilage has been removed together with a malignant tumour. The condition must be distinguished from oedema or pressure from haemorrhage. The treatment is by intubation and, if necessary, tracheostomy.

Diagnosis of these complications is difficult. A safe guide would be that if respiratory obstruction occurs after thyroidectomy sufficient to prevent the patient from sleeping, then intubation or tracheostomy is indicated.

Nausea can also be troublesome during recovery unless anti-emetics have been prescribed or included in the anaesthetic technique.

Thyroid 'crises' are seldom encountered with modern treatments. When they occur delirium, restlessness, tachycardia and sweating are the prominent signs. Treatment is by cooling, digitalis, and antithyroid drugs as recommended by the patient's physician, who should always be called in consultation.

## 42.3  Mastectomy

The main hazard of mastectomy, whether local or radical, is blood loss during the operation from oozing afterwards.

Passage of an endotracheal tube is by no means essential but is helpful during radical mastectomy, because more room becomes available for surgeons and assistants. A long acting relaxant is preferable for intubation to prevent straining during the positioning for surgery. It also allows controlled respiration with halothane which, aided by a modest foot-down tilt, lowers blood pressure, provides good venous drainage, and reduces bleeding. During the preliminaries a careful watch on the blood pressure is needed since in the absence of surgical stimulus systolic pressure can fall steeply requiring a reduction of halothane concentration. The stimulus of the surgical incision ensures a substantial rise. An intravenous drip (although not necessary for simple mastectomy) should be routine for the radical procedure during which blood loss should be measured and accurately replaced, together with a further quantity for that (not measured) on the towels and gowns, and the loss from postoperative oozing. At least two units of blood are necessary.

## 42.4  Bilateral Adrenalectomy

Bilateral adrenalectomy with bilateral ovariectomy is undertaken for multiple metastases arising from carcinoma of the breast.

Patients are always in poor physical condition, emaciated with pleural effusions and painful metastatic deposits in bones. X-rays should be studied pre-operatively to determine the presence of metastases and of pleural effusion, which if sufficient to cause breathlessness should be aspirated before anaesthesia, but otherwise after induction to reduce discomfort and distress.

Cortisone cover is essential before and after operation: 100 mg one hour before operation and four hourly the first operative day, eight hourly the second, decreasing progressively to a maintenance dose of 25 mg/day.

Deficiency of cholinesterase (related to multiple metastases) may reduce the duration of action of non-depolarising relaxants.

Care is needed when positioning patients on the table to avoid pathological fractures due to bony metastases or skin damage at pressure points due to absence of subcutaneous fat.

At first sight, surgery on such patients may appear to impose an unjustifiable strain but subsequent relief of pain and the remission of growth that follows is adequate compensation.

### 42.5  Thymectomy

Thymectomy is undertaken to relieve myasthenia gravis, unfortunately not always with success. The operation is rare. It involves splitting the sternum and risk of opening both pleural cavities.

Assessment and care of patients with myasthenia gravis is discussed in Chap. 5. Considerable blood loss may occur during this operation and hence generous provision should be made for replacement of fluids lost during the procedure as well as afterwards by oozing. Patients receive neostigmine as part of their treatment and this gives rise to excess mucus secretion which will require suction during the operation and intermittent injections of atropine.

### 42.6  Carcinoid Syndrome (Argentaffinoma)

Carcinoid is a rare tumour of primitive embryological cells, which secrete humoral substances, usually serotonin and bradykinin. They are very small tumours and are found commonly in the appendix and small bowel. They are orange in appearance and have been called argent-affinomata.

Clinical features include flushing (rather like the menopause), looseness of the bowels and bronchial spasm. Valvular lesions of the heart and hypertrophy of its muscle also occur. Symptoms are not usually severe, unless metastases are present in the liver, when serotonin has more opportunity to reach the peripheral circulation, resulting in exacerbation of symptoms, especially those of the cardiovascular and respiratory systems. Patients usually receive drugs which block the peripheral effects of serotonin, one such is 1-methyl-D-lysergic acid butanolamide maleate (Deseril) 2 mg three times a day. Chlorpromazine also antagonises serotonin and could be useful as a pre-operative or premedicant drug.

During anaesthesia serotonin may produce rises in blood pressure, tachycardia, increase in gut motility, rise in blood sugar and prolonged recovery.

Many anaesthetic drugs are said to intensify these effects, since they stimulate secretion of serotonin or bradykinin. Such drugs include morphine, suxamethonium, curare, gallamine and alcuronium, halothane and catecholamine vasopressors.

In these circumstances patients should receive good sedative pre-medication, but omitting opium alkaloids, induction should be smooth and spraying of the nose with local analgesic before intubation is advisable. There is no objection to maintenance of muscle relaxation with pancuronium, continuing anaesthesia with nitrous oxide and oxygen, supplemented by the neuroleptanalgesic drugs, fentanyl or phenoperidine.

# 43 Endoscopy

Endoscopy has been mentioned in the section dealing with ear, nose and throat surgery but oesophagoscopy and bronchoscopy and associated hazards can conveniently be discussed in this chapter.

There are few anaesthetic procedures in which cooperation and understanding between anaesthetists and surgeon are more vital to safety than laryngoscopy, bronchoscopy and oesophagoscopy. Both operators are in competition for access to the upper air passages. Success depends entirely on the anaesthetist providing the endoscopist sufficient space and time whilst ensuring the patient remains unconscious and motionless and receives sufficient oxygen. Hazards in these procedures arise from the equipment used, the anaesthetic method and the physical state of the patient.

## 43.1  Equipment

Before inducing anaesthesia, surgeons should be asked to check their equipment. Lighting systems can be a source of bother unless fibrelight equipment is available. When dependent on bulbs, transformers or batteries and connecting flexes, pre-anaesthetic checking to ensure they are in working order is essential. Spare bulbs should be available and an alternative source of light in case a battery fails at a vital moment. Older types of illumination with bulbs also carry danger of fire and explosion and exclude use of cyclopropane or ether.

Suction apparatus with suitable suction ends must be available as well as biopsy forceps of correct size. Attention to these preliminaries beforehand allows completion of the procedure without delay and reduces risk to a minimum.

## 43.2 Anatomical Difficulties

Patients often present anatomical difficulties, e.g. awkwardly placed or crowded dentition or expensive fragile bridge work, especially of the upper incisors. These create considerable difficulty when inserting a rigid oesophagoscope or bronchoscope. Arthritis affecting the thoracic and cervical vertebrae and kyphoscoliosis also make practical difficulties and sometimes make the procedure impossible. A calcified vertebral artery is liable to kink after hyperextension of the neck, so that conscious patients may faint or stop breathing. In a paralysed ventilated patient the effect on breathing is missed, until respiratory failure or delay in recovery suggests that a cerebrovascular accident has occurred.

## 43.3 Bronchoscopy

Bronchoscopy can be performed satisfactorily with topical analgesia as well as under general anaesthesia.

### 43.3.1 Topical Analgesia

Topical analgesia is safer and has no particular time limit, but is unpleasant for patients. It is less employed since short-acting relaxants have allowed provision of improved conditions for surgeons and a pleasanter experience for patients. It is possible that the amnesic properties of diazepam revealed during its use for gastroscopy may resurrect an interest in topical methods for bronchoscopy.

The mouth, fauces and pharynx are rendered insensitive by a spray of 4% lignocaine. Thereafter either: (a) an injection of 2 ml 10% cocaine or 4% lignocaine is made through the cricothyroid membrane; or (b) 10 ml doses of 10% lignocaine aerosol spray are directed through the vocal cords with the aid of a mirror or by means of a laryngeal syringe with the tongue held forward. All patients should be instructed not to drink or eat anything for three hours after application of topical analgesia.

### 43.3.2 General Anaesthesia

As already mentioned, general anaesthetic techniques for laryngoscopy and bronchoscopy do not differ materially though for topical methods 2% lignocaine spray of the pharynx and larynx is all that is needed for laryngoscopy. The aim of all methods of general anaesthesia is to secure oxygenation of patients whilst the airway is occupied by a bronchoscope or laryngoscope.

For short diagnostic procedures, pre-oxygenation before induction with thiopentone followed by 50 mg suxamethonium gives approximately 3-5 min for the endoscopist to visualize the bronchial tree. When the patient needs more oxygen, the anaesthetist asks the surgeon to occlude the end of the bronchoscope to allow insufflation of oxygen and 1% halothane through the side-piece. In addition to cyanosis, indications for additional oxygen are slowing or irregularity of the pulse.

For longer procedures, some mechanical means of injecting nitrous oxide and oxygen is often used. The Sanders injector for oxygen only is an American device. In England successful trials have been carried out with an Entonox injector which directs jets of 50% nitrous oxide and 50% oxygen through a fine catheter.

There are also apnoeic oxygenation techniques. After induction (as already described) supplementary doses of suxamethonium ensure patients remain apnoeic, whilst oxygenation is achieved either by insufflation of oxygen at high flows through a tube or catheter lying alongside the bronchoscope or placed there beforehand, or through the side arm of the bronchoscope, which is not as effective, especially if the end of the bronchoscope is in one of the main bronchi thus oxygenating only one side. The success of this technique depends on the fact that oxygen enters the bloodstream from the alveoli faster than release of carbon dioxide. If the bronchial tree is kept full of oxygen, patients remain well oxygenated although the $P\text{CO}_2$ may rise slowly (about 0.44 kPa/min).

Patients are said to remain apnoeic and in good condition for up to 15 min. With rising carbon dioxide, arrhythmias are likely to occur and sinus tachycardia is common so a careful watch should be kept on the pulse for signs of carbon dioxide accumulation (bounding pulse) as well as disturbances of cardiac rhythm.

Unless a substantial dose of thiopentone has been given, i.e. 500 mg for an adult, a 'top-up' dose of 0.1 mg should be given every 10 min to make sure that consciousness does not return.

### 43.3.3  Complications

Complications (other than respiratory) during bronchoscopy are rare.

The most alarming is haemorrhage following biopsy. If an artery is punctured a blocker or endobronchial tube should be passed. This emergency poses great difficulties for beginners and even in experienced hands is often fatal.

### 43.3.4  Recovery

Postoperatively, the lateral position during recovery is essential to allow blood and secretions to flow out through the mouth. Contra-indications to bronchoscopy include any respiratory obstruction, and copious sputum. As bronchoscopy is usually a diagnostic procedure there appears little point in performing it on cachectic and moribund patients.

## 43.4  Oesophagoscopy

Full muscle relaxation is essential during oesophagoscopy in order to position the head to the best advantage and to relax the cricothyroid sphincter. Induction is usually with thiopentone followed by 100 mg suxamethonium to obtain maximum relaxation. For intubation, a nylon-reinforced flexible cuffed tube should be used. The cuff should only be inflated with the least amount of air needed to give an airtight fix because overinflation can interfere with passage of the oesophagoscope. Oesophageal suction is essential for this purpose, especially to remove any collection of fluid above a stricture. Possible complications are rupture of the oesophagus followed by mediastinitis and haemorrhage from trauma, biopsy or distended veins.

Injection of sclerosing fluid into dilated veins in patients with advanced cirrhosis of the liver is performed through an oesophagoscope. Patients are often in partial liver failure and have already had severe haemorrhage, with the stomach containing swallowed blood. As liver function is depressed by opiates premedication should be avoided. A good intravenous drip is essential. Coughing and straining must be avoided and respiration should be controlled throughout the procedure by a combination of muscle relaxants and halothane. As the surgeon needs uninterrupted access whilst injecting veins all anaesthetic connections between the patient and the anaesthetic apparatus, i.e. the tube, catheter mount and anaesthetic hoses should be checked for security so that movement of the oesophagoscope does not disconnect them. It is usual to dim the theatre lights during the procedure but as the patients are in poor physical condition there should be a separate source of light for anaesthetists (e.g. a small torch) to check the oxygen supply and the presence of cyanosis. If a cardioscope is not in use a finger should always be kept on the patient's pulse throughout.

## 43.5  Gastroscopy and Colonoscopy

### 43.5.1  Gastroscopy

Gastroscopy has become a commonplace procedure and for elective examination most gastro-enterologists are satisfied with the amnesic properties of intravenous diazepam supplemented by a small intravenous dose of an opiate. Pentazocine (Fortral) is popular, for no other reason than that it is not subject to D.D.A. regulations and is therefore easily obtainable without the fuss and bother over keys and signature that always accompanies the modest request for 50 mg pethidine; pethidine is, however, preferable since it avoids bizarre and unpleasant side-effects of pentazocine and is cheaper.

Some surgeons prefer general anaesthesia for gastroscopy, which they often carry out prior to laparotomy for haematemesis in order to exclude bleeding oesophageal varices. Cannulation of bile and pancreatic ducts also is usually carried out under general anaesthesia.

### 43.5.2  Colonoscopy

Most operators ask for general anaesthesia for this procedure which can be carried out under spontaneous respiration with no need for endotracheal intubation.

### 43.5.3  Perforation

The main hazard of these procedures is perforation of stomach or bowel, which may only be detected during recovery when patients complain of abdominal pain with tenderness and muscular rigidity on abdominal examination.

# 44 Radiological Departments

## 44.1 Working Conditions and Facilities

In many radiological departments the anaesthetic hazards due to poor facilities for induction, for technical support, and for recovery are often as great as those involved in the procedure itself.

The fault does not necessarily lie with radiologists or their staff, but in the fact that when most radiological departments were constructed, the use of general anaesthesia was not even contemplated nor was the purchase of anaesthetic apparatus included in the budget.

Hence the anaesthetic apparatus is usually old, taken out of service from the local operating theatres where it has been replaced by more modern equipment.

Storage for drugs, tubes, syringes and laryngoscope is unsatisfactory. They are usually kept either in a cupboard in the corner of the X-ray room or scattered all over the apparatus.

A technician or nurse assistant is not usually available nor is there any recovery area.

Usually a nurse from the ward (not necessarily experienced) is asked to supervise the recovery of the patient in a corridor; the nurse will generally resist the urging of the radiological staff to remove the patient until completely satisfied recovery is complete.

Radiological screening is a constant feature of a radiological anaesthesia which takes place in dim light or total darkness. Anaesthetists should insist on having some means of illuminating gas flows and observing the presence and absence of cyanosis in their patients.

Exposure to radiation is by no means negligible and in spite of protective clothing, no monitoring is ever taken of the anaesthetist. This is surprising, bearing in mind the attention that has been directed and the massive literature that has accumulated about theatre contamination, whose harmful effects still remain largely hypothetical, although those of radiation are well known.

This dismal picture is a warning not to expect too much when visiting X-ray departments for anaesthetic assignments. One should arrive early in order to prepare drugs and tubes and check apparatus, tubes and laryngoscopes (always insist on having two) before beginning induction of the patient.

## 44.2 Indications

Anaesthesia is required mainly for neuroradiology and vascular procedures. Indications for anaesthesia vary according to the availability of trained staff and the fortitude and emotional stability of the patient. Procedures where discomfort exceeds pain, e.g. myelograms, are usually performed under some tranquillising or opiate combination except where emotional instability or problems of communication make this impossible.

## 44.3 Angiography

Carotid and vertebral angiograms are performed for diagnosis of intracranial lesions and examination of abdominal, iliac, femoral and popliteal arteries in circulatory deficiency of the lower limbs. Other arteries examined are the renals, for renal disease, and branches of the abdominal aorta, for hepatic and splenic lesions.

### 44.3.1 Approaches
The approach to the carotid artery is percutaneously in the neck and hence endotracheal intubation is necessary, preceded by spraying of the vocal cords and trachea with lignocaine, which together with maintenance of anaesthesia with halothane reduces incidence of coughing and straining, which can displace the needle in the carotid artery. Coughing is also likely to occur when changing from AP to lateral views (not necessary with modern equipment). Plethoric subjects and heavy smokers can with advantage receive a small injection of suxamethonium before this manoeuvre to allow control of respiration during the changeover. If for any reason the anaesthetist finds difficulty in endotracheal intubation, it is better to abandon the procedure that day, so that preparations can be made in the radiological department for nasal intubation, which requires preliminary spraying of the nasal passages with a vasoconstrictor 20 min before intubation, to reduce bleeding. It would be most unwise to attempt this manoeuvre in a radiological department on a patient whose nasal mucosa had not been vasoconstricted, because the haemorrhage could be quite copious and

give rise to so much difficulty that the procedure would have to be abandoned anyhow.

The approach to all other arteries including the vertebral is by means of long catheters with flexible tips to facilitate entry into the artery under examination. They are usually inserted through the femoral artery. Endotracheal intubation is therefore not necessary unless the radiologist requires apnoea during film exposure (often for renal arteries) when need for paralysis by a relaxant and controlled respiration will make intubation preferable.

### 44.3.2  Complications of Arteriography

Patients requiring carotid vertebral angiography often have central nervous lesions, which of themselves can contribute to neurological complications. Temporary paresis from vascular spasm and more permanent lesions from atheromatous emboli are said to be commoner after vertebral angiography.

On recovery severe nausea and headache are often experienced. An analgesic and anti-emetic should be prescribed in case such symptoms do occur.

Haematomata at the site of femoral or carotid puncture may form, unless pressure is maintained for at least 10 min after withdrawal of needle or catheter.

### 44.4  Air Encephalography

The introduction of the EMI scanner has largely replaced the investigation of air encephalography. Whilst it is possible to carry out this procedure under sedation without a general anaesthetic, it is extremely unpleasant for the patient and impossible where for reasons of temperament or language patient co-operation is not possible.

Hazards of anaesthesia for this procedure arise from the many positions required and the possible effects on systolic blood pressure—a hazard which it has in common with myelography. Indeed, in anaesthetising for either of these procedures, the anaesthetist is constantly required to break the rules of good anaesthetic practice by moving the patient in a short time from a steep head-down tilt to a steep foot-down tilt.

For encephalography, the patient is placed in a sitting position in a special chair after induction with the head bent forward in much the same position as that described for neurosurgery of the posterior fossa (see Chap. 34). Maintenance of anaesthesia is best carried out with spontaneous respiration under nitrous oxide, oxygen and ½ to 1% halothane. A reliable method of measuring blood pressure is indispensable, as for neurosurgery. Provided a light plane of anaesthesia can be maintained, patients tolerate the many changes of position remarkably well.

Postoperatively, severe headache is experienced with nausea which may respond favourably to 50 mg chlorpromazine intramuscularly. There is also some general cardiovascular depression and patients give the impression of severe exhaustion (which is not surprising).


## 44.5 Myelography

Myelography consists of insertion of radio-opaque dye into the subdural space with the patient in the prone position, after which films are taken in steep head-down and head-up positions and hence the same problems of hypotension confront anaesthetists as with air encephalography. More often than not this procedure is carried out under local analgesia. General anaesthesia is reserved for patients who by reason of temperament or language cannot co-operate with the radiologist. After induction and intubation, with thiopentone and a short-acting relaxant, muscle relaxation must be maintained sufficiently long to place the patient in the prone position and apply the restraining harness to prevent sliding off the X-ray table during tilting. In these circumstances 50 mg suxamethonium is not sufficient and supplementary doses may be necessary through a previously inserted butterfly needle, which must be secured carefully so that it does not come out or perforate the vein during movement of the patient. A more satisfactory plan (especially in large patients), is to maintain relaxation with pancuronium or curare.

Postoperatively, headache and nausea are very common and are best treated as described for air encephalography. Patients should always be instructed to remain flat for 24 h after this procedure. The headache of course arises from the same causes as for spinal analgesia and the treatment does not differ (see Sect. 17.4.9).

# 45 Cardiac Departments

Most procedures for which anaesthesia is required in the cardiac department also involve the use of X-ray equipment so that the hazards set out for radiological departments generally apply with equal force in the cardiac department.

## 45.1 Cardiac Catheterisation

The purpose of cardiac catheterisation is to estimate the extent and nature of changes in the heart produced by congenital defects in children or acquired defects in older subjects. Pressure and oxygen saturation are determined in each chamber of the heart on the right and left sides. The right side is approached by means of a catheter passed from a peripheral vein. The same catheter can often be directed into the left side through a defect in the interventricular septum, or through a specially shaped needle passed through the interventricular septum. If this is not possible a separate catheter is passed up an artery and through the aortic valves into the left side of the heart.

As all patients have abnormal hearts, cardiac irregularities and cardiac arrests are real hazards and the procedure is sometimes fatal.

Patients can be divided into three groups: (a) infants and young children with congenital defects; (b) adults with valvular defects of rheumatic origin, often endocarditis, and (c) adults with arteriosclerotic defects. The proportion of patients is roughly equal, but in some clinics children predominate. Mortality of the procedure is higher in infants and lower in adults. The overall rate was 0.5% in one series, but the rate for young children was five times higher than that of teenagers and adults.

The procedure is intended to measure cardiac performance at rest.

This requires what is called 'steady state of anaesthesia', during which there should be no variations in blood flow, blood pressure or oxygen saturation.

### 45.1.1  Anaesthetic Requirements

Although it is possible to carry out this investigation under sedation, many centres prefer general anaesthesia. There is no agreement about the best method and over 42 techniques have been described. Whatever method is used success will depend on the following:

1) Absence of depression of cardiac function

2) No change in respiration, heart rate or blood pressure for two hours, thus precluding intermittent doses of respiratory depressants, or changes in concentration of inhaled anaesthetics

3) In case of emergency, rapid recovery, making inhalational techniques preferable to intravenous methods

4) No increase of myocardial irritability, which cuts out cyclopropane (which in any case is precluded because of its explosive properties)

### 45.1.2  Sedation Techniques

Combinations of opiates and tranquillisers produce minimal physiological disturbance and allow patients to breathe air, but their effects are unpredictable and supplementary doses may be required, with unwelcome variations in respiratory function and blood oxygen tension.

### 45.1.3  General Anaesthesia

Intravenous induction is followed by intubation and then (after resumption of spontaneous respiration) maintenance with a set concentration of an inhalational agent can continue for an indefinite period. High concentrations of oxygen must be avoided; some authorities recommend air as a vehicle for the inhalational agent, the most popular of which is halothane. Whatever method is used complications arise from disturbance of rhythm or even ventricular fibrillation, hence a continuous ECG monitoring of cardiac function is essential.

*Ketamine.* Ketamine has been used successfully in small children and infants for cardiac catheterisation. Although there is a preliminary rise in arterial pressure it subsides before the vital measurements are made. (See Sect. 12.3.5 for further details concerning ketamine.)

## 45.2  Angiocardiography

Angiocardiography may be performed during cardiac catheterisation or as a separate procedure. Vagal inhibition is a possibility and continuous ECG recording is essential. Radio-opaque sodium acetrizoate is injected very rapidly into a large vein as a bolus to reach the heart and great vessels. There may be a pause in respiration during the procedure, as well as coughing, bronchospasm and laryngospasm. When performed after cardiac catheterisation under sedation, general anaesthesia is essential. There is no restriction of oxygen consumption however, but apnoea is essential during exposure of X-ray film.

### 45.2.1 Complications

In addition to disturbances of cardiac rhythm, infants may suffer significant blood loss during these procedures after multiple samplings of blood, and because electric warming devices interfere with X-ray activity and cannot be used, infants may become hypothermic, unless the radiological room is kept at a reasonable temperature. Sensitivity responses following injection of dyes are rare and respond to anti-histamines or steroids.

## 45.3  Pacemakers

Patients requiring pacemakers suffer from impaired conduction of nerve impulses down the bundle of His and have a pulse rate below 50, unaffected by exercise or vagolytic drugs. From time to time the heart fails to beat at all causing sudden black-out, sometimes resembling an epileptic fit (Stokes-Adams syndrome). To improve conduction small electrical pacemakers are inserted into the chest or abdominal wall, from which wires are threaded through the diaphragm or chest wall into the left ventricle to ensure regular contraction.

The hazards of anaesthesia include asystole and fibrillation. The presence of an assistant is helpful, to keep a watch on the ECG tracing and assist in any resuscitation measures which may become necessary. Before starting anaesthesia patients should be asked whether they have had steroid therapy, as this form of treatment is sometimes recommended to improve the cardiac condition.

Premedication should be with atropine only. If a pacemaker has not previously been inserted the anaesthetist should ask for insertion of a temporary pacemaker in the left atrium if possible.

Standard endotracheal anaesthesia with topical anaesthesia of the trachea and spontaneous respiration is a suitable method.

During insertion and testing of the device, no muscle relaxant should be used as it would obscure painful muscle twitches arising from false positioning of the pacemaker.

Although there is no blood loss an intravenous infusion is necessary to allow the introduction of isoprenaline to increase heart rate if necessary.

When it is not possible to insert a temporary pacemaker, thiopentone induction should be omitted, because a sudden fall of systolic blood pressure in patients with fixed cardiac output may cause myocardial ischaemia, through reduction of coronary flow.

Patients with pacemakers tolerate surgery well, provided the surgeon is warned not to use diathermy, which damages the pacemaker and renders it inoperative. Even with pacemakers, output is still fixed and care should be taken to maintain full oxygenation and replace accurately any blood loss during the procedure.

*Cardioversion.* Cardioversion is a procedure undertaken to reverse atrial fibrillation and consists of application of a sharp electrical shock to the precordium. Although it is quickly accomplished, it is too painful to undertake without anaesthesia.

Thiopentone alone is often sufficient, supplemented if necessary by nitrous oxide and oxygen. No complications have so far been recorded.

# 46 Day Surgery

Medical administrators favour day surgery because it reduces waiting lists and overall costs of treatment by avoiding occupation of a bed intended for acute illness. Because of these advantages, funds often become available for setting up day surgery units. Often, however, staffing requirements do not receive proper consideration, especially those for anaesthesia. Anaesthesia for day surgery is not simple and cannot be left in the hands of those with little training or experience. It often presents difficulties requiring as much anaesthetic skill as major procedures. There should therefore always be an anaesthetist responsible for the anaesthetic services in a day unit, and attendance there should be included as part of the training of junior staff.

## 46.1 Equipment

Unless a consultant is responsible, day units are likely to receive old, substandard equipment no longer used in operating suites, such as old-fashioned Boyle's bottles for vaporising halothane, inaccurate rotameters and cylinder yokes. In addition to up-to-date anaesthetic apparatus, the equipment must include laryngoscopes, endotracheal tubes, suction and all facilities for treatment of cardiac arrest. A circular sent out by the Department of Health and Social Security dealing with this aspect, states, 'It is essential that the quality of hospital services required for day patients should be of an equivalent standard to that provided for "in patients" and this includes equipment.'

## 46.2  Preparation of Patients

All patients selected for day surgery should ideally receive a pre-anaesthetic examination in the outpatient department when their appointment is made. A medical check-up for every patient is essential. Usually up to 10% are under treatment for hypertension or some other complaint, having been prescribed antihypertensive drugs, beta-blockers, steroids, digitalis and frusemide. Others, particularly those requiring check cystoscopies, may be heavy smokers and suffer from chronic bronchitis.

All patients should receive typewritten instructions to refrain from food or drink for at least 4 h before anaesthesia, to arrange for a friend or relative to accompany them on their homeward journey, and not to drive an automobile. Investigations show that about 2% ignore dietary instructions, while many more ignore instructions about returning home.

## 46.3  Premedication

Day patients do not usually receive premedication, on the grounds that it would delay recovery. However, a high incidence in some patients of after-effects which are related to the anaesthetic has given rise to a change in attitude. A drying agent is certainly necessary, and can always be included with an intravenous induction agent.

Opiate premedication reduces the amount of inhalational anaesthetic required to suppress reflex movement, and by the same action may often render inhalational supplements after intravenous induction unnecessary. No evidence exists to show whether intramuscular opiates would extend the time needed before safe discharge from the unit. It is possible that this would not be greatly prolonged (a) because less of the other more powerful inhalational agents would be needed and (b) because opiates, although they cause light-headedness similar to that following half a glass of spirits, do not have hypnotic properties or cause loss of balance.

Apprehensive patients should be prescribed a mild sedative to take 1 h before arriving at the unit, or on arrival, and be asked to rest for half an hour. Diazepam 5-10 mg or phenobarbitone 1 mg is suitable.

## 46.4  Consent Forms

An addition to the customary items, the consent form should include confirmation by the patients that, as instructed:
 1) They have not taken food or drink within 4 h
 2) They undertake not to drive or operate machinery for 24 h
 3) They will not consume any alcohol for 24 h

## 46.5 Technical Hazards

Compared with premedicated subjects, intravenous anaesthesia without premedication is associated with an increase in spontaneous movement of the limbs, hiccup, coughing and laryngospasm.

Except for short procedures like orthopaedic manipulation, supplementary nitrous oxide and oxygen, and an inhalational agent, trichloroethylene or halothane, can reduce these side-effects provided the airway is kept clear and some carbon dioxide is added to inhaled mixtures to deepen respiration and thus increase blood concentration of the inhalational agent.

Every effort must be made to keep a clear airway by holding the jaw forward, for insertion of an airway at too light a plane can cause gagging, coughing and laryngospasm.

Intravenous diazepam should be used with great caution in day surgery units. Full recovery from its effects takes longer than recovery from general anaesthesia. Patients may appear normal, but still be amnesic and subject to psychomotor disturbance.

## 46.6 Recovery

Recovery facilities in day surgery units are just as necessary as for long-stay patients in respect of space, staff and equipment.

Many patients experience undesirable side-effects after recovery. Questionnaires, with a reply rate as high as 90%, show positive answers in 80% of females and 50% of males. One out of four experiences drowsiness, giddiness, nausea or headache. The incidence is related to the length of the procedure, especially if it exceeds 15 min. Halothane increases the incidence of headache. Since opiate premedication reduces the amount of halothane required, it might also lessen the incidence of headache.

Dental procedures are associated with a high incidence (77%) of after-effects. The use of an endotracheal tube is bound to increase incidence of sore throat, and suxamethonium used as a relaxant will give rise to muscle pain. It is interesting to note, however, that in one series where the patients did not receive suxamethonium just over 30% complained of muscle pain.

Nausea and vomiting occur more often after dental anaesthesia, but patients find this less distresssing than headache, drowsiness and dizziness. Dental patients probably require more analgesic than those who have undergone minor surgical procedures. All patients should receive the option of some pain-killing sedative before setting out on their homeward journey.

## 46.7 Return Home

Despite the use of informative leaflets, many patients fail to make arrangements for somebody to accompany them home, and a fair number do not even refrain from driving an automobile. In one report, 31% returned home unaccompanied and 9% drove their own automobile, although experiencing headache, drowsiness and dizziness.

## 46.8 Conclusion

Anaesthesia for day surgery is by no means free from hazards, and the incidence of unpleasant side-effects is unacceptably high. Attempts to introduce short-acting intravenous agents with rapid recovery have not proved totally satisfactory. Sensitivity to alphaxalone and alphadolone, which can be fatal, has been reported, whilst spontaneous muscle movement under etomidate interferes with surgery unless the patients receive opiate premedication. This objection to etomidate will of course be weakened if it can be shown that opiate premedication does not delay recovery and reduces unwelcome side-effects, as suggested in Sect. 46.3.

Greater use of regional and local blocks is an obvious way of making day surgery less hazardous and more pleasant for the patients.

# Selective Bibliography

Detailed references have been intentionally omitted from the text. A splendid collection of anaesthetic references can be found in Atkinson and Rushman's *A Synopsis of Anaesthesia* continuing the pioneering work of J. Alfred Lee (Atkinson RS, Rushman GB (1977) A synopsis of anaesthesia, 8th edn. John Wright, Bristol). I have used that work freely during the preparation of this book and would advise seekers of further knowledge to consult it when they find no references here.

Part I  *Pre-operative Assessment, Medicolegal and Occupational Hazards*

## 2  Cardiovascular Disease

Kyei-Mensah K, Somanathan S (1976) Medical disease and the anaesthetist. Proc R Soc Med 69:731-736

Prys-Roberts C (1976) Medical problems of surgical patients: hypertension and ischaemic heart disease. Ann R Coll Surg Engl 58:465-472

## 4  Haematological Disorders

Howells TH (1976) Anaesthesia and blood diseases. In: Hewer CL, Atkinson RS (eds) Recent advances in anaesthesia, vol 12. Churchill Livingstone, Edinburgh London, pp 120-130

Howells TH, Huntsman RG, Boys JE, Mahmood A (1972) Anaesthesia and sickle cell haemoglobin. With a case report. Br J Anaesth 44:975-987

Oduro KA, Searle JF (1972) Anaesthesia in sickle-cell states: a plea for simplicity. Br Med J IV:596-598

## 8  Medicolegal Hazards

Simpson K (1977) The anaesthetist and the law. 18th John Snow memorial lecture. Anaesthesia 32:626-635

## 9  Occupational Hazards

Smith WDA (1976) Pollution and anaesthetist. In: Hewer CL, Atkinson RS (eds) Recent advances in anaesthesia, vol 12. Churchill Livingstone, Edinburgh London

Walts LM, Forsythe AB, Moore G (1975) Critique: occupational disease among operating room personnel. Anesthesiology 42:608-611

Part II   *Considerations Relevant to All Procedures*

**10   Preparation and Use of Anaesthetic Apparatus**

Adams AP, Henville JD (1978) anaesthetic circuits and flexible pipelines for medical gases. In: Hewer CL, Atkinson RS (eds) Recent advances in anaesthesia, vol 13. Churchill Livingstone, Edinburgh London, pp 23-55

American National Standards Institute. Standard Z 79-8 (1979) Minimum performance and safety requirements for components and systems of continuous flow anesthetic machines for human use

Department of Health and Social Security. Health technical memo-randum No. 22 (Supplement March 1977). Permit to work system for piped medical gases, medical compressed air and medical vacuum installations

Newton NI, Adams AP (1978) Excessive airway pressure during anaesthesia: hazards, effects and prevention. Anaesthesia 33:689-699

**11   Fires, Explosions and Electric Shock**

Dobbie AK (1969) The electrical aspects of surgical diathermy. Biomed Eng 4:206-216

Editorial (1979) Nothing can be made fool proof, because fools are so ingenious. Anaesthesia 34:145-146

**12   Induction**

Clarke RSJ, Dundee JW, Garrett RT, McArdle GK, Sutton JA (1975) Adverse reactions to intravenous anaesthetics: a survey of 100 reports. Br J Anaesth 47:575-585

Evans JM, Keogh JAM (1977) Adverse reactions to intravenous anaesthetic induction agents. Br Med J II:735-736

Hart SM, Fitzgerald PG (1975) Unexplained jaundice following non-halothane anaesthesia. Br J. Anaesth 47:1231-1236

Simpson BR, Strunin L, Walton B (1971) The halothane dilemma: a case for the defence. Br Med J IV:96-100

Strunin L, Simpson BR (1971) Halothane in Britain today. Br J Anaesth 44:919-924

**15   Positioning Patients for Surgery**

Martin JT (1978) Positioning in anesthesia and surgery. Saunders, Philadelphia

**16   Maintenance of Anaesthesia**

Hopkin DAB (1961) Some suggestions for the neural basis of the anaesthetic state. Br J Anaesth 33:114-118

Hopkin DAB (1963) Some recent views on the mechanisms of conscious-ness and the differences between the central actions of anaesthetics and some of the newer sedative agents. Proc R Soc Med 56:981-983

Magoun HW (1963) The waking brain, 2nd edn. C Thomas, Springfield (Ill.)

## 17 Local Analgesia

Dawkins CJM (1969) An analysis of the complications of extradural and caudal block. Anaesthesia 24:554-563
Lee JA, Atkinson RS (1978) Sir Robert Macintosh's lumbar puncture and spinal analgesia: intradural and extradural, 4th edn. Churchill Livingstone, Edinburgh London

## 18 Cardiovascular Hazards

Ashton H (1963) Critical closure in human limbs. Br Med Bull 19:149-154
Burton AC (1951) On the physical equilibrium of small blood vessels. Am J Physiol 164:319-329
Burton AC (1965) Haemodynamics of circulation. In: Ruch V, Patton HD (eds) Physiology and biophysics, 19th edn. Saunders, Philadelphia, pp 523-542
Burton AC, Yamada S (1951) Relation between blood pressure and flow in human forearm. J Appl Physiol 4:329-339
Jennings AMC (1964) Some observations of critical closing pressures in the peripheral circulation of anaesthetized patients. Br J Anaesth 36:683-693
Nelson TE, Flewellen EH (1979) Rationale for dantrolene vs. procainamide for treatment of malignant hyperthermia. Anesthesiology 50:118-122
Nichol J, Girling F, Jerrard W, Claxton EB, Burton AC (1951) Fundamental instability of the small blood vessels and critical closing pressures in vascular beds. Am J Physiol 164:330-344
Relton JES, Britt BA, Steward DT (1973) Malignant hyperpyrexia. Br J Anaesth 45:269

## 19 Controlled Hypotension

Bodman RI (1967) Controlled hypotension. In: Hewer CL (ed) Recent advances in anaesthesia and analgesia, vol 10. Churchill, London, pp 90-117
Leigh JM, Millar RA (1975) Symposium on deliberate hypotension in anaesthesia. Br J Anaesth 47:743-810
Tinker JH, Michenfelder JD (1976) Sodium nitroprusside: pharmacology, toxicology and therapeutics. Anesthesiology 45:340-354

## 20 Intravenous Therapy and Central Venous Pressure Lines

Allsop JR, Askew AR (1975) Subclavian vein cannulation: a new complication. Br Med J IV:262-263
Walters MB, Stranger HAD, Rotem CE (1972) Complications with percutaneous central venous catheters. JAMA 220:1455-1457

### 21  Blood Transfusion

Department of Health and Social Security, for National Blood Transfusion Service (1975) Notes on transfusion

### 23  Cardiac Arrest

Feldman S, Ellis H (1975) Principles of resuscitation, 2nd end. Blackwell, Oxford

### 24  Intensive Care

Gilston A (1976) Facial signs of respiratory distress after cardiac surgery: a plea for the clinical approach to mechanical ventilation. Anaesthesia 31:385-397


Part III  *Emergency Surgery*

### 25  Stomach Content

Norton-Perkins HD (1974) Conduction analgesia. In: Thornton HL, Norton-Perkins HD (eds) Emergency anaesthesia, 2nd edn. Arnold, London, pp 129-179

Thornton HL (1974) Preoperative assessment and preparation of the patient. In: Thornton HL, Norton-Perkins HD (eds) Emergency anaesthesia, 2nd edn. Arnold, London, pp 1-9

### 26  Shock: Vascular Responses to Injury, Haemorrhage and Infection

Hopkin DAB (1977) A common neural basis for shock states and suggestions for treatment by regulation of afferent input to the central nervous system. In: Vasconcelos G (ed) Proceedings—6th World Congress of Anaesthesiology. Excerpta Medica, Amsterdam (International Congress Series 387, pp 368-371)

Livett BG (1973) Histochemical visualization of peripheral and central adrenergic neurones. Br Med Bull 29:93-99

Simmons RL, Ducker TB, Martin AM, Anderson RW, Noyes HE (1968) The role of the central nervous system in septic shock: I. Pathologic changes following intraventricular and intracisternal endotoxin in the dog. Ann Surg 167:145-157

Smith AD (1973) Mechanisms involved in the release of noradrenaline from sympathetic nerves. Br Med Bull 29:123-129

Ukai H, Moran WH, Zimmermann B (1968) The role of the visceral afferent pathways on vasopressin secretion and urinary excretory patterns during surgical stress. Ann Surg 168:16-28

Vogt H (1973) Functional aspects of the role of catecholamines in the central nervous system. Br Med Bull 29:168-171

Wilmore DW, Long JM, Mason AD, Pruitt BA (1976) Stress in surgical patients as a neurophysiologic reflex response. Surg Gynecol Obstet 142:257-269

Part IV   *Individual Types of Procedure*

### 31   Operative Obstetrics

Green RA (1978) Anaesthesia for caesarian section. Anaesthesia 33:70
Steel GC (1978) Personal view. Br Med J I:1049

### 34   Neurosurgery

Hunter AR (1975) Neurosurgical anaesthesia, 2nd edn. Blackwell, Oxford

### 36   Paediatric Surgery

Rees GJ (1960) Paediatric anaesthesia. Br J Anaesth 32:132-140

### 37   Dental Surgery

Green RA, Coplans MP (1973) Anaesthesia and analgesia in dentistry. HK Lewis, London

### 44   Radiological Departments

Campkin TV (1976) General anaesthesia for neuroradiology. Br J Anaesth 48:783-789
Royal Society of Medicine (1975) Anaesthesia in the x-ray department. Proc R Soc Med 68:765-766

### 46   Day Surgery

Burn JM (1979) A blueprint for day surgery. Anaesthesia 34:790-805
Routh GS (1979) Day care surgery under general anaesthesia in a purpose built unit. Anaesthesia 34:809-822

# Index

# Disaster Medicine

Editors: R. Frey, P. Safar
Sub-Editors: P. Baskett, K. Stosseck,
P. Sands, J. Nehnevajsa

Technological advances in industry, trans-
portation and armaments have increased
the risk of mass injury and death far beyond
that hitherto posed by natural forces alone.
The medical profession thus finds itself confronted with the need for a new dimension
in such events, namely "disaster resuscito-
logy." This is best described as the role
critical care medicine – resuscitation, emergency care and intensive care – plays in
attending to individual survivors to reduce
the number of deaths and longterm injuries
in the wake of disaster.
In cooperation with the Club of Mainz on
Emergency and Disaster Medicine World-
wide, the Springer Series on Disaster Medicine concentrates on the importance of critical are in disaster relief. It provides an international forum for discussion of not only the
medical and organizational aspects of
disaster response, but also the social, psychological and ecological effects such events
bring with them. Each volume will focus
on specific disaster problems, as, for
example, cold and frost injuries, nuclear
accidents, and air and rail crashes.

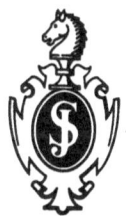

Springer-Verlag
Berlin
Heidelberg
New York

Volume 1

## Types and Events of Disasters Organization in Various Disaster Situations

Proceedings of the International Congress
on Disaster Medicine, Mainz 1977
Part I
Editors: R. Frey, P. Safar

1980. 97 figures, 33 tables. XX, 355 pages
ISBN 3-540-09043-6

**Contents:** Types and Events of Disasters.
Definition of Disasters. – Organization in
Various Disaster Situations (Local, Region-
al, National. – Workshops: Global
Disaster Situations. Local/Regional
Disaster Situations. Definite Care in
Disaster Situations.

Volume 2

## Resuscitation and Life Support in Disasters Relief of Pain and Suffering in Disaster Situations

Proceedings of the International Congress
on Disaster Medicine, Mainz 1977
Part II
Editors: R. Frey, P. Safar

1980. 81 figures, 52 tables.
Approx. 320 pages
ISBN 3-540-09044-4

**Contents:** Resuscitation and Life Support
in Disasters. – Relief of Pain and Suffering
in Disaster Situations. – Workshops: Resus-
sitation. Intravenous Fluids. Relief of Pain
and Suffering. Free Topics. – Conclusion.

# Acute Care

Based on the Proceedings of the Sixth International
Symposium on Critical Care Medicin
Editors: B. M. Tavares, R. Frey
1979. 133 figures, 97 tables. XVI, 345 pages
(Anaesthesiology and Intensive Care Medicine,
Volume 116)
ISBN 3-540-09210-2


C. Burri, F. W. Ahnefeld

# The Caval Catheter

With the collaboration of K. H. Altemeyer, B. Gorgass,
O. Haferkamp, D. Heitmann, G. Krischak, P. Lintner,
A. Ott, H. H. Pässler, E. Plank, D. Spilker, W. Stotz
Translated from the German Edition "C. Burri,
F. W. Ahnefeld: Cava Katheter"
1978. 54 figures, 18 tables. VII, 84 pages
ISBN 3-540-08566-1


# Clinical Management of Mother and Newborn

Editor: G. F. Marx
1979. 30 figures, 44 tables. XIV, 274 pages
ISBN 3-540-90373-9


# Critical Care Medicine Manual

Editors: M. H. Weil, P. L. DaLuz
1978. 73 figures, 48 tables. XXIV, 371 pages
ISBN 3-540-90270-8


# Enzymes in Anesthesiology

Editor: F. F. Foldes
With contributions by A. A. Aszalos, F. F. Foldes,
L. C. Mark, S. H. Ngai, R. W. Patterson, J. M. Perel,
S. F. Sullivan, L. Triner, E. K. Zsigmond
1978. 34 figures, 18 tables. XIX, 368 pages
ISBN 3-540-90241-4


W. S. McDougal, C. L. Slade, B. A. Pruitt, jr.

# Manual of Burns

Medical Illustrators: M. Williams, C. H. Boyter,
D. P. Russell
1978. 214 colored figures, 4 tables. X, 165 pages
(Comprehensive Manuals of Surgical Specialties)
ISBN 3-540-90319-4

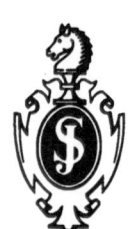

Springer-Verlag
Berlin
Heidelberg
New York